D1014668

MEDICARE

MEDICARE

Jennie Jacobs Kronenfeld

Health and Medical Issues Today

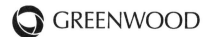 GREENWOOD

AN IMPRINT OF ABC-CLIO, LLC
Santa Barbara, California • Denver, Colorado • Oxford, England

Copyright 2011 by Jennie Jacobs Kronenfeld

All rights reserved. No part of this publication may be reproduced, stored in a
retrieval system, or transmitted, in any form or by any means, electronic, mechanical,
photocopying, recording, or otherwise, except for the inclusion of brief quotations in a
review, without prior permission in writing from the publisher.

Library of Congress Cataloging-in-Publication Data

Kronenfeld, Jennie J.
    Medicare / Jennie Jacobs Kronenfeld.
        p. ; cm. — (Health and medical issues today)
    Includes bibliographical references and index.
    ISBN 978–0–313–36405–1 (hard copy : alk. paper) – ISBN 978–0–313–36406–8
(e-book)
1. Medicare. I. Title. II. Series: Health and medical issues today.
[DNLM: 1. Medicare. 2. Health Care Reform—United States. 3. Insurance, Long-Term
Care—United States. 4. Medicare–history. WT 31]
RA412.3.K757   2011
368.4′2600973—dc22   2010038267

ISBN: 978–0–313–36405–1
EISBN: 978–0–313–36406–8

15 14 13 12 11   1 2 3 4 5

This book is also available on the World Wide Web as an eBook.
Visit www.abc-clio.com for details.

Greenwood
An Imprint of ABC-CLIO, LLC

ABC-CLIO, LLC
130 Cremona Drive, P.O. Box 1911
Santa Barbara, California 93116-1911

This book is printed on acid-free paper ∞

Manufactured in the United States of America

Contents

SERIES FOREWORD

Every day, the public is bombarded with information on developments in medicine and health care. Whether it is on the latest techniques in treatment or research, or on concerns over public health threats, this information directly affects the lives of people more than almost any other issue. Although there are many sources for understanding these topics—from Web sites and blogs to newspapers and magazines—students and ordinary citizens often need one resource that makes sense of the complex health and medical issues affecting their daily lives.

The *Health and Medical Issues Today* series provides just such a one-stop resource for obtaining a solid overview of the most controversial areas of health care in the 21st century. Each volume addresses one topic and provides a balanced summary of what is known. These volumes provide an excellent first step for students and lay people interested in understanding how health care works in our society today.

Each volume is broken into several sections to provide readers and researchers with easy access to the information they need:

- Section I provides overview chapters on background information—including chapters on such areas as the historical, scientific, medical, social, and legal issues involved—that a citizen needs to intelligently understand the topic.
- Section II provides capsule examinations of the most heated contemporary issues and debates, and analyzes in a balanced manner the viewpoints held by various advocates in the debates.
- Section III provides a selection of reference material, such as annotated primary source documents, a timeline of important events, and

a directory of organizations that serve as the best next step in learning about the topic at hand.

The *Health and Medical Issues Today* series strives to provide readers with all the information needed to begin making sense of some of the most important debates going on in the world today. The series includes volumes on such topics as stem-cell research, obesity, gene therapy, alternative medicine, organ transplantation, mental health, and more.

PREFACE

Medicare is the best-known federally funded program that provides health insurance to large numbers of Americans. Medicare was passed in 1965 and has become one of the best-known programs of the U.S. government, along with Social Security, that provides income support for the elderly. For those age 65 and over, the Social Security legislation, which passed in the 1930s during the Great Depression and impacted a large number of U.S. citizens in the 1940s through 1960s, is one of the most used and discussed federal programs. The same is true for Medicare which provides health care insurance to pay for the health care services of most U.S. elderly, as well as to some disabled people in the United States.

For many U.S. citizens, as they turn 65, one of their most important actions to secure their future access to health care is to apply for their Medicare card, just as applying for Social Security benefits is also an important step towards securing their economic future. In most major U.S. political campaigns since 1965, the continuance of both Medicare and Social Security is seen as essential to secure the votes of the elderly. This holds true for the votes of many younger U.S. citizens, since many have parents or other older relatives who rely upon these programs for their basic economic support and access to health care.

How did Medicare become such an important and large program, and how well has it worked in the past for its beneficiaries? What are the current problems and issues that need to be resolved for Medicare to continue its important role in meeting the health care needs of the elderly? These are some of the questions to be addressed in this book. The above description might convince you that there is a broad consensus about the importance of Medicare in our country, and that is what led to the initial passage of the legislation. You might also think that the presence of a broad consensus is important whenever changes to the program are discussed by politicians. In actuality, the idea of a broad consensus about Medicare is more complicated. There was controversy at the time of the initial debates that led to the final passage of the program. In addition, there have been controversies about some aspects of Medicare ever since the program was passed, especially once it became clear that its costs were higher than the initial projections. And these controversies continued as concerns have increased about the rising costs of Medicare, along with the rising costs of medical care and health insurance in general. In addition, there are controversies about what changes are needed for the program in the future to secure its continuation.

Some of the controversies today continue to relate to the cost of Medicare while others relate to deficits in coverage or services that many people assume are covered when they retire but have never been covered in much depth, such as long-term care services. Other controversies relate to the ever-increasing number of Medicare recipients and the recognition that this number will increase dramatically in future years as the large baby boomer generation begins to age. This growth will dramatically increase the overall costs for the program, even if the costs per participant are controlled. These are some of the issues to be addressed in this book.

The aforementioned are debates about the program as a large government program, its sources of funding, and its stability from these funds. These are ways to look at policy from a macro- (or large scale) perspective. Other ways to look at a program such as Medicare are from the perspective of the individuals enrolled in the program, the micro-perspective. While this book will focus upon the larger-scale macro issues, it is important to realize that some of the controversies about Medicare also grow from the micro-level experiences of individuals. For example, when the elderly have trouble paying for their health care expenses and they are using Medicare to cover these expenses, they become angry with the program. They tell their adult children about their frustrations, and, if frustrated enough, they might even write or call their legislators to complain about the program. These are ways, in a democracy, in which micro-level issues can rise to be part of the macro-level public debate over policies.

This book will help you to understand the history of Medicare, some of the current issues with the program, other government-funded health care programs, and also provide ideas to think about in terms of potential changes of the program. Because of the passage of health care reform in March 2010, and its impact upon Medicare policy, there will continue to be important changes in Medicare now and in the future. Many of the more important changes in that legislation begin slowly, with major changes starting in 2014. However, some changes to Medicare begin more quickly, starting in 2010, such as changes in the drug program (Part D) and the elimination of copayments and deductibles for certain preventive services. The new legislation is also aimed towards reducing deficits in the Medicare Trust Fund, but it is too soon to know its full effectiveness.

This book is part of the *Health and Medical Issues Today* series, and follows the general series approach of being divided into three major sections. Section I (Chapters 1–3) provides historical information about U.S. health care before Medicare and the debate over the passage of the program, information about the early use and costs of Medicare, and important changes and expansions to the program such as coverage for people with kidney problems and modifications in how hospitals and physicians are paid. These chapters will cover the first 35 years of the Medicare program.

Section II (Chapters 4–5) covers major current issues, beginning with the prescription drug coverage addition to Medicare, and discusses other topics such as Medicare and HMOs and the lack of long-term care coverage in any depth by Medicare. This section also includes information about the other two large government programs to provide health care services, Medicaid and SCHIP (State Child Health Insurance Program). Medicaid provides health care coverage for the poor and there are some important ways that it may often be combined with Medicare for some elderly. SCHIP was the newest addition to large federal health insurance programs, prior to the 2010 health care reforms, and provides health insurance coverage to the children of the working poor.

Section II also includes more detailed discussion of the demographic-based funding crisis and issues linked to the retirement of the large baby boom generation, and a discussion of potential changes that are expected to occur in Medicare as the result of the 2010 health care reform. They are really reforms of the health insurance market rather than the creation of a new federal health program such as Medicare, or a joint federal-state program such as Medicaid and SCHIP. This new legislation will, however, also encompass important changes to the programs of Medicare and Medicaid.

Section III of the book provides annotated primary sources about the Medicare program prior to the 2010 reforms, a timeline of important developments and changes in the Medicare program, and selected resources and sources for further information.

SECTION I

Overview

CHAPTER 1

The History behind the Passage of Medicare

On July 30th, 1965, in Independence, Missouri, former President Harry S. Truman's hometown, President Lyndon B. Johnson signed the legislation that created the Medicare program. He picked this location to sign the passage of the bill to honor former President Truman and his failed efforts to pass major health legislation (with a program with many similarities to Medicare being proposed). This symbolic moment reflects what most people who have written and studied about Medicare and its initial passage in the United States agree was the end of a long period of attempts to pass major health care legislation in the United States. The two major amendments to the Social Security legislation, Title XVIII and Title XIX, were signed into law and became the federal Medicare program that provides health insurance coverage to most of the elderly in the United States and the federal-state funded and administered Medicaid program that provides health insurance coverage to many of the poor in the United States.

While these were both innovative programs within the U.S. context, the idea of government providing health insurance to its citizens had been discussed in the United States since the early 1900s. By 1965, most European countries had enacted some form of major health insurance for many of its citizens. Often these efforts in many European countries began with the poor or laborers, and then expanded to cover more of the population. There were many times within the 20th century, prior to the 1960s, when the issue of the role of the government in health care in the United States was raised. Some of the issues were more generally seen as part of income support policies rather than health care specifically. Some of the major concerns about the role of the federal government in health care concerned the government's role in medical research, funds for hospital construction, as well as the direct provision of services to people, either through government programs or government-funded health care insurance.

A nation's health policy is part of its overall social policy, and this is true when examining the Medicare program in the United States. Therefore, both the formulation of health policy and social policy are influenced by a variety and array of social and economic factors. Factors such as the nature and history of existing social institutions, ritualized methods for dealing with social conflict, and the general goals and values of a society all play a role in the formulation of social policy. In addition, important overall ideological factors are inseparable from the basic ideological orientation of the United States. Two of the most important aspects of ideological orientation in the United States are the economic system of capitalism and the philosophy of classical liberalism or individualism. The United States is a capitalist country, and has often viewed it best if most issues can be handled through the private marketplace, rather than through government. Liberalism or individualism emphasizes individuals as the basis and justification for the creation of government. Most of the things affecting individual well-being, including health care, are to be both the choice and the responsibility of the individual. This was certainly the approach to government in the United States up to around 1900, except in times of major political crises such as the Civil War. Only in the 20th century, has the U.S. government been viewed as a counterweight to other powerful forces in the society and the provider of last resort for certain types of services. Government began to be regarded as the provider of public goods, services for overall well-being which in earlier times had been provided by the private marketplace.

The issue of government pensions to provide economic security to Americans did not begin with Social Security, but rather with efforts to reward veterans of various wars. While the first national pension program for soldiers passed in early 1776, prior even to the signing of the Declaration of Independence, the larger war pension program related to Civil War veterans. The Civil War Pension program began during the Civil War, with the first legislation in 1862 providing for benefits linked to disabilities that were a direct consequence of military duty. Widows and orphans were eligible to receive pensions equal in amount to that which would have been payable to the deceased solider if he had been disabled. In 1890, the link with service-connected disability was broken, and any disabled Civil War veteran could qualify for benefits. By 1906, old age became a sufficient qualification for benefits. By 1910, over 90 percent of the remaining Civil War veterans were receiving benefits under this program (Historical Background and Development of Social Security, 2009). This was not just a small program that gave benefits to a few people, but, in terms of the U.S. government budget, a major program. In 1894, military pensions accounted for 37 percent of the entire federal budget. Thus, America had a pension program in place prior to the passage of Social Security that did provide some help with economic security to some parts of the population. This did not include health or sickness insurance, however.

By the time of the Great Depression in the 1930s, however, the number of people still receiving Civil War pensions had declined greatly, and there were many public calls for some type of new program to deal with the economic crisis. In 1932, President Franklin D. Roosevelt (FDR) introduced his economic security proposal based upon social insurance rather than upon welfare assistance. This changed the terms of the debate in the United States, as it was no longer a choice between radical changes and old approaches that did not work. The "new" idea of social insurance, an idea already widespread in Europe, became an innovative alternative. Social insurance, as conceived by FDR would address the permanent problem of economic security for the elderly by creating a work-related, contributory system. Workers would provide for their own future economic security through taxes paid while employed. This created an alternative both to reliance upon welfare and to radical changes in our capitalist system.

There had been some previous attempts prior to the Great Depression for large-scale social insurance programs in the United States including health-related provisions. The first major attempt occurred during the Progressive Era in the United States, when Americans realized that countries such as Germany were the first to provide compulsory sickness insurance for their workers in 1883. England began a limited program for workers in 1911. In 1912, former President Theodore Roosevelt, addressing the convention of the Progressive Party, issued a call for social insurance that included sickness insurance. His third-party run for the presidency was not successful, however. Private groups were also pushing for some type of sickness insurance at that point in time, especially the American Association for Labor Legislation (AALL), a group started in 1906 that included academic social scientists, labor leaders, and lawyers. This group was successful in pushing states to adopt workmen's compensation legislation, and planned a focus on medical care insurance as a next step, employing a state-by-state campaign approach. The group expected success, especially when the American Medical Association (AMA), the main organization of physicians in the United States at that point, initially supported the proposals. The AALL did manage to have the legislation introduced in 15 state legislatures and to have commissions formed to study health insurance in 10 states, but little actual legislation was ever passed. By 1920, any momentum for compulsory health insurance had stalled. Also, by 1920, more conservative elements within the AMA became active in the leadership of the group and realized that local medical societies were opposed to state health insurance bills. In 1920, the AMA formally declared its opposition to plans of compulsory medical insurance whether controlled or regulated by a state or by the federal government.

By the time World War I ended, the push for any type of sickness or health insurance had stalled in a variety of ways. As previously mentioned, the AMA was formally opposed to the idea. The association of Germany as an enemy country tainted the idea of sickness insurance among some parts of the U.S. public. Another factor that created a negative image for compulsory sickness or health insurance was the Communist takeover of Russia following the Russian Revolution in 1917 as compulsory health insurance was one program of the Communist Party in Russia. In addition, private insurance companies and pharmaceutical companies opposed the idea, as did some parts of the American labor movement, especially the American Federation of Labor (AFL) under Samuel Gompers. Historians have argued that Gompers' fear that compulsory social insurance would be an excuse for government control of working men was an important reason why the United States did not follow the example of countries such as England that insured its lower-paid workers and the working class against illness.

The 1920s in the United States were not a time of much social experimentation, especially in terms of federal programs, both in welfare and in health. About the only major expansion in the health arena that passed in the 1920s was the Sheppard-Towner Maternity and Infancy Protection Act of 1921. The Act provided a system of federal funding to enhance the health and welfare of women and children. Grace Abbott, Julia Lathrop, and other feminist activists worked to get the statute adopted, and it was consistent with the social goals of the women's movement of the 19th century, and many attributed its successful passage to the passage of the Women's Suffrage Amendment. Various medical groups, including the American Medical Association, opposed this passage and continued to oppose the program, so that funding under the Act ended in 1929, and the effort to achieve further federal support of such programs was not successful until the New Deal. It was the crisis of the Great Depression that brought renewed discussion of these topics.

SOCIAL SECURITY LEGISLATION AND OTHER ATTEMPTS IN THE 1930S AND WWII

President Franklin Delano Roosevelt was in favor of social security legislation, both as a reaction to the Great Depression and as part of a political climate that favored greater federal activism. A committee on economic security was created by FDR in 1934 with the mission of drafting a program of social insurance legislation, including health insurance. Given the depths of the Depression, many experts were focused upon the need for unemployment assistance and old-age insurance. A work-related, contributory system was often the focus of discussion for old-age insurance. The original Social Security Bill did contain a line to authorize a study of health insurance. The AMA learned of this line, and was very opposed to this part of the legislation. Many negative telegrams were received about this part of the legislation, leading the Ways and Means Committee to unanimously remove the line from the bill, so that it did not endanger the passage of the rest of the legislation. FDR also feared that the controversy over the issue of government health insurance might jeopardize both the overall Social Security Bill and his chances of reelection.

One impact of this brief attempt to include health insurance in the Social Security legislation was that the AMA reversed their opposition to private health insurance. The AMA began to endorse Blue Cross hospital plans, as well as some commercial hospital insurance plans. They also supported the creation of state Blue Shield plans to cover physician expenses, and actually encouraged the development of these plans, which did help to cover bills in a doctor's office.

Within Congress and among social and health policy experts, the success of Social Security in providing income protection to dependent women and children, the blind, and the aged led to continued interest in the topic of health insurance (the name that now was used for what had formerly been described as sickness insurance coverage). Senator Wagner from New York introduced a national health bill into Congress in 1939. By 1943, national health insurance legislation was introduced into Congress in most years, often sponsored by Wagner, Senator Murray from Montana, and Congressman Dingell from Michigan in the House of Representatives. This new legislation was broader in scope than the Progressive Era attempts, and wanted coverage of all Americans, not just industrial workers. Given the focus on World War II, and the costs of that war, these attempts never succeeded and were never formally endorsed by FDR. With the death of FDR in 1945, and the ending of the war later that year, the focus upon new plans for social and health policy shifted to President Harry S. Truman and what became known as his "Fair Deal" proposals.

THE FAIR DEAL AND EFFORTS FOR UNIVERSAL HEALTH PROPOSALS

President Truman began with a broader, more expansive view of health insurance. While the initial proposal to examine health insurance as part of the Social Security legislation was viewing health insurance as an income protection approach, the Fair Deal proposals initially viewed health insurance as a remedy for inequitable distribution of, and access to, medical care services. Early discussion in the Truman administration focused upon the importance of access to and use of health care services being determined by a person's need for care and their illnesses, rather than their income. The minimal access to health care services through charitable clinics and doctors was not enough in this approach. Truman became the first U.S. President to formally endorse national health

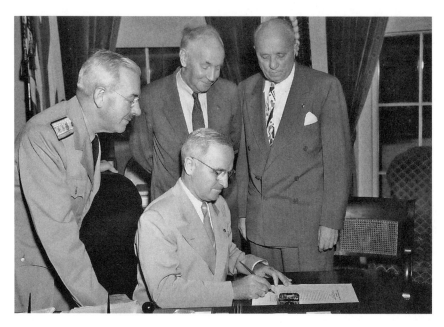

President Harry S. Truman signs a health bill in Washington, D.C., on August 8, 1946. The bill authorizes federal agencies and departments to establish health programs for their employees. Looking on are, from left to right: Dr. Thomas Parran, surgeon general of the Public Health Service; Harry B. Mitchell, president of the Civil Service commission; and Watson B. Miller, Federal Security Agency administrator. (AP Photo)

insurance legislation. He endorsed the Wagner-Murray-Dingell Bill and pushed for its enactment in 1948, although nothing happened that year, a year in which Congress became known as the "do-nothing Congress." In the election that followed, Truman argued against how little the Congress had gotten accomplished and this argument became an important part of his election victory.

When Truman won the 1948 presidential election, he again pushed for the enactment of his national health insurance program. The plan was quite comprehensive, covering all medical, dental, hospital, and nursing care expenses. It would be a contributory plan for most workers, and cover the worker and dependents, with federal grants to the states for those who were destitute and not working. The financing mechanism was a 3 percent payroll tax, to be divided equally between employee and employer. To try to blunt criticism that the government was taking over medicine, doctors and hospitals would be free to join or not join the plan and patients would be free to choose their own doctors. Doctors who participated would be paid for their services through the creation of a national hospital board.

Even though public opinion initially seemed favorable and President Truman was supportive, the legislation did not pass. The reaction in Congress was disappointing and complex. The Democrats had gained

75 seats in the House of Representatives, but there were a group of anti-Truman southern Democrats that linked with Republicans to block this bill (and much of the rest) of Truman's domestic agenda. Another major opposition group was organized medicine, who managed to link the issue with Cold War fears of socialism and linked the proposals to socialized medicine, raising fears among the public and lowering the support for the proposals. The AMA launched the most expensive lobbying campaign in U.S. history up to that point and used this campaign to label supporters of the Truman plan as socialists. In addition, the AMA labeled the plan as one which would hurt the quality of medical care by providing control over medicine to the government. The AMA allied with groups such as the Chamber of Commerce that opposed a government health insurance program and private insurance companies including Blue Cross. The success of the AMA in the defeat of this proposal led to the organization being viewed as the most powerful interest group in the United States. Moreover, the AMA continued their opposition by defeating at least three congressmen in the 1950 elections who had been supportive of the health insurance proposals.

At the time of the defeat of Truman's national health insurance proposal in 1949, there was talk about resubmitting the proposal. Some form of the Murray-Wagner-Dingell Bill continued to be introduced into Congress for many years, even though there was almost no chance of it being discussed seriously or passed. By the time of the 1950 midterm elections in which Democrats and supporters of national health insurance lost seats in Congress, it was clear that Truman's time to pass such a plan had come and gone. Truman persisted in requesting compulsory health insurance legislation in 1950, 1951, and 1952, and lambasted the AMA for their campaign against "socialized medicine" and their characterization of his health insurance plans as socialism. This had little real political impact. Although Democrats held a majority in both the House of Representatives and the Senate after the 1948 election, the political strength of a conservative coalition of southern Democrats and Republicans made the passage of much of Truman's social agenda unlikely, and this was certainly true in the health arena. Truman's absence of a programmatic majority in the Congress meant that controversial proposals (and compulsory health insurance coverage was very controversial) had no chance of being enacted.

A SHIFT TO THE ELDERLY

Among strategists for health insurance, the level of controversy over compulsory health insurance was a problem. People such as Wilbur J. Cohen and Isadore S. Falk who were very involved in the early drafting of health insurance proposals as part of Social Security and who were very involved in drafting President Truman's health insurance proposals, started to think of other strategies. Cohen and Falk served as advisers to Federal Security Agency administrator Oscar Ewing. Together, they all came up with the idea of switching attempts to have reform in health care and health insurance to more modest, narrower proposals. They decided that a plan more likely to pass Congress was one that tried to provide federal health insurance to beneficiaries of Social Security payments as part of the Old Age and Survivors Insurance. In June 1951, Ewing announced a limited proposal to provide 60 days of health insurance each year to the then seven million elderly retirees receiving Social Security benefits, but this did not pass.

The decision to shift to a plan focused upon the elderly is an interesting decision, and one that by the 1960s leads to the creation of Medicare and to treatment of health care for the elderly as one type of program, in contrast to health care for the poor, or health care for everyone. This was clearly a political, pragmatic decision. In a comparative context, it is an unusual decision, because most other industrial countries in the world had not begun their programs with the aged. More typical has been the coverage of low-income workers, but this has involved means-tests to be sure that the people benefitting were low-income people, and, from the Roosevelt era on, the assumption has been to try and avoid the stigma of means test in the United States. A focus upon the aged is part of an incremental approach to reform of the health care system in the United States. Many policy analysts and political scientists have pointed out that, in the United States, rather than having large major public policy shifts, changes in public policy often come in small increments. The shift to a focus on the elderly reflects the success of this incremental approach in the United States.

According to two researchers who have studied the debates around the creation of Medicare, Marmor (2000) and Oberlander (2003), there were four major objections to the Truman health plan that any modified strategy of health insurance needed to meet to have a chance of political success. These objections were first, that general medical insurance would be a "give-away" program and would lack distinction between the deserving and undeserving poor; secondly, that it would aid too many wealthy or well-off Americans who did not need the aid; thirdly, that utilization of existing medical services would grow too rapidly and exceed the capacity of the system; and lastly, that there would be excessive federal control of physicians and this could provide a precedent for socialism in the United States. To get around these objections, the idea of a program for the elderly was attractive. Through a restriction of beneficiaries to the elderly, the concern about a giveaway program was diminished, because the elderly were seen as a group that was, on average, poorer, sicker, and less likely to be insured as compared to other Americans. In addition, the aged garnered public sympathy as a group, and the issue that a person should simply earn more money to pay for the service was not a relevant consideration. By this time in the United States, many people were receiving health insurance through their workplace, but, as people grew older and retired, they lost this insurance, making the restriction to the elderly a logical one based on the way health insurance was growing in the United States.

Once the major idea for health reform became a program for the elderly, the decision to tie a program to the existing Social Security system made sense based upon the widespread support among the public. One advantage was that the Social Security system was not viewed as a welfare benefit but as an earned benefit of retired workers, since it was funded by people who had paid into the system through their payroll taxes. This idea that the benefits had been earned, as opposed to being a welfare program, was very important in gaining the support of the public. Because it benefited the majority of the elderly, support could be gathered among a wide range of current workers, both as a benefit they would receive in the future and one that would benefit their parents more quickly. Thus, it was hoped, a shift to a program for the elderly would gain broad political support. However, during the Eisenhower administration (1952–1960), most Medicare bills, whatever the type, really had no chance of being enacted. In 1952, President Eisenhower had campaigned against socialized medicine, which for him included both the earlier Truman proposals and more modest proposals for health insurance for the elderly. In addition, in 1952, the Republicans gained majorities in both the House of Representatives and the Senate, and there was a general conservative shift in the national political mood.

ACTIVITIES PRIOR TO THE MEDICARE DEBATE OF THE 1960S

Although the 1950s were generally a more conservative era, they were not static. In 1954, the Democrats regained control of both Houses of Congress, raising the chances of more discussion of various social policy issues. However, the prospects for a Medicare-type proposal were not good, since the Democrats still did not have a programmatic majority capable of enacting federal health insurance for the aged. The leadership in both the House Ways and Means Committee and the Senate Finance Committee were resistant to a Medicare proposal, which, along with the absence of a president supportive of the legislation, made a major political change unlikely.

Slowly, some change began to occur. In 1956, disability insurance for workers over the age of 50 was passed, an approach that was championed by people such as Wilbur Cohen, director of research for the Social Security Administration, along with people who had been important in the Truman years in developing the plans for national health insurance. They saw the disability legislation as another incremental achievement that helped to provide some greater security for older workers in the absence of national health insurance. In 1957, Representative Aime Forand, a Democrat from Rhode Island, proposed a bill on Medicare. Beginning in 1958, serious Congressional interest in special health insurance programs for the elderly began to grow. From 1958 to 1965, the congressional finance committees held annual hearings on the topic. In 1958, the Ways and Means Committee in the House held a hearing on the bill, but the new Democratic chair of the committee, Wilbur Mills from Arkansas, opposed the Forand Bill and it did not make it out of committee.

These hearings did revitalize Medicare as a political issue, and brought back the attention of the AMA, who had believed they had defeated these ideas for good during the Truman administration. In response, the AMA raised their lobbying budget fivefold to increase their ability to criticize and raise opposition against the Forand Bill. Bringing back the arguments from the late 1940s, the AMA argued that the Forand Bill would bring an unwelcome intrusion of the government into private medical practice. They also argued that the elderly were financially better off than some other age groups, but the main thrust of their opposition was ideological. They wanted to convince the public that health insurance for the elderly would be the first step to national socialism, using code words of the time that were designed to raise political concerns and make many politicians reluctant to support the idea. The AMA also helped line up other opponents, some, such as the American Hospital Association, the National Association of Blue Shield Plans, and the Life Insurance Association of America with some focus on health care or insurance concerns as well as various business organizations such as the National Association of Manufacturers, the Chamber of Commerce, and the American Farm Bureau Federation. Given the ideological orientation of the opposition, groups such as the American Legion also opposed the legislation.

Despite the hope among the advocates of health insurance for the elderly that a move to enact government health insurance only among the elderly and tie it to the existing, popular Social Security program would dampen political opposition, this did not happen initially. The acrimonious debate at the time of the Truman proposal reappeared, with similar proponents and opponents, and public attention was redrawn to the issue as political commentators and the press began to follow parts of the debate. Among the proponents of the legislation were major labor groups such as the AFL-CIO, health-related groups such as the American Nurses Association, the National Association of Social Workers, and the American Geriatrics Society and more liberal social-action oriented groups such as the Council of Jewish Federations and Welfare Funds, the American Association of Retired Workers, and the National Farmers Union. The splits between the groups in opposition to and in favor of Medicare were often also splits on other important political issues of the day, such as disability insurance and federal aid to education. Gradually, however, the shift to a focus upon the elderly and the creation of lobby groups representing the elderly did begin to shift some of the terms of the debate.

A special Senate subcommittee on aging was created, under Democratic Senator Pat McNamara from Michigan, and the group held a series of public meetings on the topic in 38 different cities between 1959 and 1961. This raised the public consciousness of issues of the elderly generally, and especially the issue of health insurance for this demographic group. An interesting split occurred between the Forand Social Security approach and a welfare-oriented approach. The Social Security approach pushed to cover all the aged who were covered under Social Security, while a welfare approach would focus on people over 65 whose own resources were inadequate to meet medial expenses. In terms of benefits, the Social Security approach covered hospitalization, nursing homes, and surgical coverage while the welfare approach was broader and covered physicians' services, dental care, drugs, as well as hospital expenses. The Social Security approach proposed funding through additional Social Security taxes, a regressive approach that takes more money from less well-paid workers, since, at that time, there was a fairly low cap on the amount of wages taxed for Social Security. (There is still a cap today on wages taxed for Social Security but at a much higher level, and there is no longer a cap for Medicare, although there was such a cap initially.)

An advantage of the Social Security approach, however, was the absence of any means test which critics felt would be insulting to the elderly. In addition to insulting the elderly, there was an argument that the absence of a means test would broaden the political appeal of the program, since it would benefit all elderly. A welfare approach would use federal income tax revenues along with state matching funds, generally a more progressive source of taxation. The Social Security approach would lead to uniform national standards administered by the Social Security Administration whereas a welfare approach would lead to varying standards administered by state and local officials. In some ways, it is surprising to realize that it was liberals who favored the Social Security approach and the more conservative welfare-backers who favored the broader benefits for a smaller group of the elderly, those financially destitute. The reason that liberals supported the Forand Bill was skepticism that a means-tested, state-administered assistance approach would actually be utilized or implemented.

Although the Eisenhower administration remained opposed to any legislation similar to the Forand Bill, some Republicans, including the likely Presidential candidate, Richard Nixon, became worried that this opposition could be a detriment to a Republican presidential candidate. Some of the Congressional conservatives, especially on the Democratic side, came up with a counterproposal, a bill sponsored by Senators Robert Kerr of Oklahoma and Wilbur Mills of Arkansas. This bill proposed expanding federal aid to states that were providing medical care assistance to the elderly poor. The Kerr-Mills Bill proposed federal matching grants of 50 to 80 percent of the costs to participating states. This was the welfare-oriented approach. By the time the bill was up for a vote in Congress, Democratic Presidential Candidate John F. Kennedy had decided to use medical care for the aged as one policy issue to distinguish himself from Nixon; this became a plank in the Democratic Party position at the nominating convention. The emphasis raised the attention being paid to the Kerr-Mills Bill, and the AMA decided to endorse the bill as a preferable alternative to Medicare itself.

The Kerr-Mills legislation was finally passed by Congress and signed by President Eisenhower. The victory was viewed differently by different groups. While conservatives viewed this as legislation passed as an alternative to Medicare, liberals viewed it as a first step towards a broader Medicare proposal. Despite some enthusiasm for the program when passed, the legislation was not very successful in practice. Although some experts had estimated that there were 2.4 million people on old-age assistance and 10 million medically indigent that could share in the program, some critics such as Senator McNamara felt many of the states would never provide the matching funds needed to participate in the program. McNamara's predictions proved more accurate over time. Many states never participated in the program (32 of 50 by 1963), and, by 1965, five large industrial states (California, New York, Massachusetts, Michigan, and Pennsylvania) were using almost 90 percent of the Kerr-Mill funds even though those states had only a third of the elderly population in the United States. Not only was the geographic distribution of the recipients limited, but the range of benefits provided was also less than allowed by the program. In 1963, only four states provided the full range of care allowed for in the bill.

THE FIGHT FOR MEDICARE LEGISLATION IN THE KENNEDY ADMINISTRATION

As previously mentioned, John F. Kennedy made the passage of Medicare legislation a plank in the Democratic Party platform for the 1960 presidential election. Kennedy's victory in that election meant that now there was presidential sponsorship for the Medicare legislation. In his first state of the union address, President Kennedy called for the enactment of health care for the elderly by the end of the year, but this did not happen. Kennedy labeled his proposed new programs the "New Frontier" and included a variety of domestic proposals within it, including health insurance for the aged. A new Medicare bill was proposed, however, introduced by Senator Clinton Anderson of New Mexico and Representative Cecil King of California. This bill provided 90 days of hospitalization coverage, 240 days of home health services, 180 days of nursing home care, and outpatient diagnostic services. It would extend these benefits to 14 million Americans over 65 and would be financed by a one-quarter of one percent increase in the Social Security taxes. The Kennedy administration did push for this legislation, with a public campaign, a series of rallies, and a nationally televised appeal in 1962. To try to limit some of the earlier opposition to such a program, Kennedy stressed that this was not socialized medicine but prepayment for health care costs with freedom of choice assured.

Some of the same issues that hindered President Truman's push for national health insurance were also problems for President Kennedy. He lacked a firm programmatic majority in Congress, and again was often frustrated by the conservative coalition of southern Democrats and Republicans in Congress. Among his own party's leadership, Ways and Means Chair Wilbur Mills still was concerned about the program and feared that its fiscal consequences would be bad for Social Security overall. Moreover, the process for the selection of the Ways and Means Committee in the House worked against expansion of social welfare issues, including Medicare for

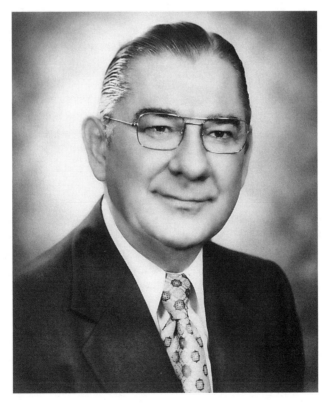

Wilbur Mills, Democratic representative from Arkansas, was a key player in the success of the 1965 Medicare bill. (Library of Congress)

the elderly. Democrats on the Ways and Means Committee in that era also composed the Committee on Committees responsible for Democratic committee assignments. This meant that the geographical distribution in the Ways and Means Committee was frozen and thus, placed the nine Democratic liberal members in a minority in terms of social policy expansions with Southern Democrats and some Republicans representing the opposition. If it was clear that the House would favor legislation, it was reported out of committee and voted on by all members. But if the senior members of this committee felt that a bill would face a bitter, closed-floor fight, typically the committee either did not report the bill out or wrote compromises into the legislation before it came to the floor of the House. Mills, whose own Kerr-Mills Bill had just become law, was not initially inclined to be supportive. Moreover, it appeared that redistricting based on the 1960 census would cause Arkansas to lose two House seats and might result in a contested election in Mills' own district, reinforcing his more conservative tendencies. Because of these pressures and the pressure from Kennedy to achieve legislative success in other areas, such as his trade and tax legislation, the Medicare Bill did not surface in 1961. No vote was even taken.

Some of the same opposing groups as were active in the Truman era again became active against a new Medicare Bill. The AMA again led the opposition, especially in terms of public advertisements and public comment. It funded newspaper, radio, and television ads that again brought out charges of socialism, arguing that a task force would enter the privacy of the examination room and eliminate the freedom of Americans to choose their own doctors and the freedom of doctors to treat patients as they saw fit. Beyond the national advertising, the AMA sponsored reproductions of congressional speeches against the bill and distributed them in many American communities and enlisted county medical societies to provide speakers against the legislation and to place material in their reading areas for patients.

Even though the Democrats retained control of Congress in the 1962 elections, not that much changed in terms of the committees controlling the introduction of legislation and the likelihood of passage of some type of Medicare legislation. While various efforts to have votes taken on the legislation did occur, nothing passed. As often happens as a presidential election begins to approach, the chances of passage in the period before the election were lower in 1963, as the Congress began to think about the elections in 1964, including the presidential election. In late November 1963, the Kennedy assassination changed many aspects of politics "as usual." Lyndon B. Johnson, the vice-president under Kennedy, took over as President and began to prepare to run for election on his own. The outcome of that election would be critical in determining the chances of Medicare passage in the future.

LYNDON B. JOHNSON, THE 1964 ELECTION, AND PASSAGE OF MEDICARE

The 1964 election produced a huge, landslide victory for the Democratic Party. Part of this was a reaction to the assassination of President Kennedy, which increased the popularity of the Democratic Party. In addition, Lyndon B. Johnson was a skillful politician with many years of experience, and the campaign that his opponent Barry Goldwater ran never captured the support of the American electorate. The Democratic Party gained 32 seats in the House of Representatives, providing the party with a two to one ratio (295 Democratic seats to 140 Republican seats), the largest lead since New Deal Days under FDR. The Senate margin was also a large one for the Democratic Party, with 68 Democratic senators and only 32 Republican senators. One reading of Johnson's victory over Goldwater was that it provided support for what Johnson called his "Great Society" programs that included Medicare as one of the pieces of social legislation. He had campaigned for a variety of social reforms, including Medicare, and emerged from the election with control over both Houses of Congress and a popular mandate for social change. Because the debate over the legislation ended up framing the resulting Medicare program, with some strengths but also some important weaknesses, understanding the debates of that time helps to understand

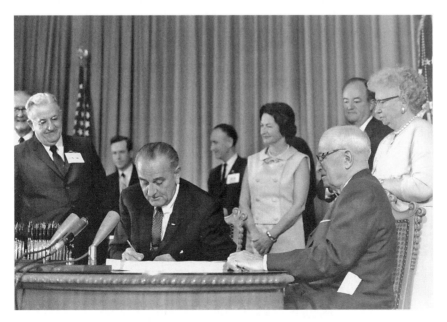

President Lyndon B. Johnson signs the Medicare program into law on July 30, 1965. On the right is former president Harry Truman, who became the first person to apply for the federal health care program. (Lyndon B. Johnson Library)

problems in Medicare in its early decades, and even some of the problems that remain today.

Using their large majorities, House Democrats made sure that delaying tactics for a variety of pieces of social legislation did not occur by preventing such tactics through modifications in the House rules. Most importantly, the 21-day rule was put back into place, meaning that bills could be discharged from the House Rules Committee after a maximum delay of three weeks. The composition of the Ways and Means Committee was also modified to reflect the strength of the parties in the House as a whole, rather than the three majority and two minority members of the past. This changed the composition of the committee in 1965 from 15 Democrats and 10 Republicans to 17 Democrats and 8 Republicans. The passage of Medicare legislation now seemed assured, and the issue became what the actual legislation would include. In some ways, as other scholars have also noted (Oberlander, 2003; Marmor, 2000), this quick shift to a guaranteed success for the legislation left proponents somewhat unprepared as to whether a more comprehensive program might be the best approach, given the legislative changes. Instead, advocates continued to press for a more incremental program that emphasized maximizing consensus on a clearly defined, but somewhat minimal, set of benefits, leaving the issues of more comprehensive benefits as an area for future expansion. Basic Medicare coverage remained focused on 60 days of hospitalization and 60 days of nursing home care, with even coverage for doctor's bills an elective part of the program. Coverage was focused upon the elderly, and financing was to occur through a social security approach.

In contrast with the Democrats, the Republicans and other opponents of Medicare legislation in the past (such as the AMA), did recognize just how much the political circumstances had changed. Republicans understood that passage of some type of Medicare legislation was now virtually inevitable, and wanted to avoid being labeled as "obstructionists." Republican criticism focused on inadequate benefits, and some Republicans, such as John W. Byrnes, the ranking Republican on the House Ways and Means Committee, proposed his own bill that would provide a voluntary program of federal payments to subsidize private health insurance for the elderly. This would be a broader program, including doctor bills and drug coverage, and using general revenues to finance the program. The AMA came up with a separate proposal, called Eldercare. This program was to be implemented by states, but would include hospital and physician coverage, as well as coverage of surgical fees and drug costs, nursing home costs, and services such as x-rays and laboratory charges. By February 1965, three different proposals were before the Congress: H. R. and S. 1 also called the King-Anderson Bill, the Byrnes Republican proposal, and the AMA Eldercare proposal.

Activities in Congress were moving forward toward passage of the Administration bill (H.R. and S. 1, the King Anderson Bill). As early as January, hearings were being held, including executive sessions in private that often indicate serious movement toward passage of legislation in Congress. Members of the AMA testified at the congressional hearings, and often raised concerns about socialized medicine. This was irritating to the committee members, and Chairman Mills ended up refusing to consult AMA representatives as the hearings and deliberations continued.

By March of that year, hearings were also planned on the Republican bill by Representative Byrnes. Republicans wanted to prevent the Democrats from taking all the credit for passage of Medicare legislation, and were also publicizing the inadequacies of the Democratic bill. Byrnes emphasized the major areas of health costs not covered by the Democratic proposal, such as doctors' bills and drug costs. He also emphasized that his bill was voluntary, with the aged free to make a decision about joining. Although the AMA was publicizing its own Eldercare plan and the problems with the Democratic bill, most of the discussion in the House was about the Byrnes proposal, not about Eldercare. The Byrnes and Democratic proposals were being presented as mutually exclusive alternatives.

As a surprise move in early March 1965, Mills started discussing some ways to combine aspects of each proposal. Up to that point in time, the head of the Department of Health, Education, and Welfare (DHEW), Wilbur Cohen had mentioned a three-pronged approach: the hospital program of H.R. 1 first, then private health insurance for physician's coverage, and then an expanded Kerr-Mills program as a "safety-net" type of program for the indigent among the elderly. Despite some fears among the more liberal Democrats that Mills might try to scuttle the entire effort, Cohen became convinced that Mill's strategy was really a way to expand H.R. 1, based upon some of the criticisms of the Republicans. While Byrnes initially was not enthusiastic about this approach, the House Ways and Means Committee in March concentrated on working out some of the combinations that might be possible.

Payments for drugs outside of hospitals and nursing homes ended up being rejected for fear of costs being too high, for example. Byrnes' financing approach of individual premium payments by current Social Security recipients for physician services was adopted. Many technical issues arose that later became important in Medicare, such as how to pay hospital-based specialists such as anesthesiologists, pathologists, and radiologists. Groups such as Blue Cross and the American Hospital Association became involved in helping to draft parts of the legislation and in answering technical questions about hospital benefits. The Medicare Bill reported to the House on March 29, 1965, included parts of the original administration bill, parts of the Byrnes benefit package, and the AMA suggestion of an expanded Kerr-Mills program. These features became part of two different amendments to the existing Social Security legislation: Title XVIII which included the hospital insurance program and some of the Byrnes extensions to cover voluntary doctor's insurance and Title XIX, an expanded Kerr-Mills program that became known as Medicaid and became an addition to the initial Medicare proposal, rather than a substitute as the AMA had suggested. Despite including some of the Republican suggestions into the bill, in the final vote of the committee, there was a straight party vote of 17 in favor and 8 opposed.

The House met to vote on the legislation, now quite long (296 pages), and members gave Mills a standing ovation for his work on drafting this legislation through the committee. Byrnes had a chance to present his alternative bill, and some Democrats actually favored that option, but the proposal to send that version forward was defeated. Instead the committee bill (now H.R. 6675), was passed, largely on party lines. Because the Senate was viewed as the more liberal of the legislative bodies, there was little concern that something would pass there, although, as usual in legislation, there are always questions about the specific details. Two questions were whether the method of paying in-hospital specialists would remain and whether there might be a move to make the program more generous, perhaps by varying the hospital deductible according to the income of beneficiaries. The Senate version did have a different payment plan for the in-hospital specialists, one the AMA vehemently opposed, and unlimited hospital care with a coinsurance provision. At this point, the legislation had to go to a conference committee (a standard practice to resolve differences between the details of a bill passed in the House of Representatives and the version passed in the Senate). The House version of paying in-hospital specialists became the final version in the bill.

Most other decisions became compromises between the House and the Senate. For example, on benefit duration, the more generous Senate version had allowed unlimited days and the House version had allowed 60 days. The final version allowed 60 days with the 40-dollar House deductible and an additional 30 days with the Senate 10-dollar coinsurance provision. On skilled nursing home coverage, the more generous Senate version that allowed 100 days with a copay of five dollars a day for each day over 20 became the conference version. For post-hospital home health days, the less generous House allowance of 100 became the final version. This revised conference version was passed by the House on July 27th, and by the Senate two days later, leading to the triumphant signing ceremony in Independence, Missouri on July 30th, 1965, the birthplace of former President Harry S. Truman.

CHAPTER 2

Early Issues and Changes in Medicare: Implementation and Costs

Chapter 1 covered the history leading up to the passage of Medicare, the debates about coverage, and other details about Medicare. This chapter will focus on the early issues related to implementation and costs, and changes to the program through 1980. Many of the early issues and concerns about Medicare set the stage for today's issues and concerns about the program. One of the most important early assumptions about Medicare was that a central goal should be to bring the elderly into the mainstream of American medicine. Thus, the program ended up looking very similar to decent health insurance coverage for a typical working American at that time. This applied to benefits, reimbursement structures, and administrative aspects of the program. Medicare resembled typical Blue Cross-Blue Shield health coverage of the period, with an emphasis on coverage for acute illness, generous payments to physicians and hospitals, and little oversight. The initial positive aspects of Medicare were that the elderly received much greater access to health care services and the medical profession was reassured that the federal government would not disrupt the normal operation of the health care system.

However, many aspects of the Medicare program changed over time. The good coverage of the 1960s became problematic coverage as private health insurance changed more easily and rapidly than did Medicare. Also, the first assumption held by most of the elderly that Medicare would take care of their health care needs with few out-of-pocket expenses was not met. Nor, in some ways, was this (erroneous) assumption intended to be met even in the beginning years of the program. The lack of oversight led to high costs, which led to the reorganization of Medicare reimbursement for both hospitals and physicians, which, in turn, eventually led to the federal government changing the ways in which the health care system operated. By 1980, cost concerns and attempts to find methods to hold down costs became two very important aspects of the program, as they would in later years as well as leading up to the present debates about health care in the United States.

The second basic assumption was that Medicare would provide all elderly with the same health insurance coverage. Whatever a person's income level was before retirement, or after retirement, everyone would participate in the same program and would have the same benefits, premiums, and cost-sharing requirements. For example, a high-income individual with a large pension, in addition to Social Security and investment income, would not pay more for Medicare than an individual whose only source of retirement income was Social Security. One positive aspect of this assumption in the early years of Medicare was strong support for the program by the elderly population, since everyone received similar benefits. Over time, this aspect of the program has changed, not so much in benefits, but in the basic payments that are charged for people to participate in some aspects of Medicare. In 1965, one reason for treating all participants the same was the widely-held principle of universalism which maintained that all citizens should receive certain basic benefits. There was also a public image that the elderly were a poorer and more dependent group in the population, and therefore, were a group that deserved government assistance. While this assumption was largely accurate in 1965, it has become less so over time. Today, the average income of people 65 and over is not that much lower than the average income of many working people. Also, some elderly have important assets in houses and other retirement funds.

A third assumption, held by those who were the architects of the basic Medicare legislation, was that Medicare was considered the beginning of government's role in health insurance, and perhaps, a first step toward a more universal health insurance system. The architects of the initial legislation and the early administrators, such as Robert Ball, a commissioner of the Social Security Administration, stated that insurance for the elderly was a fallback position from more comprehensive reform. Expansions were to be expected, perhaps by age group to cover all children, or to cover broader population groups in general. Many at the time expected a drive for more changes and expansions to the system to happen fairly quickly, but this did not occur. Debates even today continue about major changes in health insurance coverage in the United States, and there have been expansions of parts of Medicare and of Medicaid over the years, and the creation of SCHIP, the state child health insurance program, during the Clinton administration. Medicare, however, has remained the major federally administered health insurance program, with its benefits restricted to the elderly and the disabled.

One final assumption of the 1965 program was that Medicare would be a system of public health insurance, guided by the federal government. Appropriating some of today's language from health care debates, Medicare was a single-payer program. This term implies a program run by the government in which the government serves as the single payer and sets the rules for payment, rather than a program that provides the elderly with subsidies to buy private health insurance. This became the basic structure of the program despite the desire of the health insurance companies and many physicians, as discussed in the previous chapter, to have a subsidized health insurance program. Many believe that the basic structure occurred because private health insurance and the marketplace were already viewed as having failed in the provision of health insurance coverage to the elderly, thus requiring government action. Over time, the basic aspects of Medicare changed in many ways. These trends and changes only make sense after a review of issues of the early operation and implementation of Medicare through 1980 which is the focus of this chapter. Chapter 3 will begin to review some of the more important changes in Medicare from the 1980s to the 1990s.

IMPLEMENTATION AND COVERAGE ISSUES

Parts A and B of Medicare

While the celebration over the passage of Medicare was very positive in July 1965, as the implementation of the program began, the complex realities of putting into place and managing such a large program soon began to emerge. Medicare has now become the single largest payer for health care in the United States, and any program of that size will bring about a variety of concerns and issues. Some of these concerns and issues were clear from its inception. The initial creation of Medicare was one that brought about complexity partly because of the two different initial aspects of the program: Part A, the hospital insurance component (or HI) that covers certain amounts of inpatient hospital care, home care, hospice care, and care in a skilled nursing facility and Part B, the supplementary health insurance portion (or SMI). Not only do Parts A and B cover different types of services, but they also include two different financing mechanisms. Initially, eligibility for hospitalization insurance (Part A) was for all individuals ages 65 and over. By 1968, this was changed to individuals ages 65 and over who were eligible for Social Security benefits. Part A helps cover inpatient care in hospitals (including critical access hospitals and inpatient rehabilitation facilities), inpatient stays in a skilled nursing facility (not custodial or long-term care services), hospice care services (added later), and home health care services.

Part A of the program is financed by a compulsory matching payroll tax, which is now up to 1.45 percent of an employee's wages. (This is in addition to the 6.2 percent payroll tax that is deducted from an employee's paycheck to cover Social Security costs.) In both taxes, the employer must match the payment. For Medicare, this is now paid on any amount of income that a person earns, although for Social Security there is still a maximum amount of earnings that are taxed ($106,800 dollars in 2009). For each program (Social Security and Medicare), the amount paid into the system by the employee is matched by the employer. People who are self-employed have a modified payment schedule, paying more than just the individual amount for people who have employers. When Medicare began, over 19 million people ages 65 and older were initially enrolled.

While on the surface the financing of Social Security and Part A of Medicare appear very similar, the logic is quite different. In Social Security, beneficiaries receive pension payments that vary according to their earnings which relate to the taxes that are actually paid into the system. If a person earns more and pays more taxes into the system, the final Social Security payment is higher, although the benefits formula favors low wage workers. In contrast, Medicare's benefits do not use the principle of earnings-related benefits—how much health care a person receives as a beneficiary generally when retired determines the size of the benefit, not the amount a person earned while working. This more explicitly carries with it a redistributive policy impact, ensuring that low-income workers will receive the same access to government-sponsored health insurance as do more affluent workers. It is not, however, as progressive a taxing approach as if all income (not just earned income, but income from interests, rents, etc.) were taxed for the benefit. Most experts believe that it was the commitment to a social insurance approach and the programmatic experience with Social Security that led to the creation of a payroll tax as the funding mechanism for Part A of Medicare. A concern with the Part A funding mechanism is that, almost from the beginning, it has faced a projected shortfall at some point. This is certainly the case today as projections begin to take into account the declining size of the work force and the increased number of beneficiaries due to the upcoming retirement of the Baby Boom generation. Some of these issues are discussed in greater detail in Section II of the book.

One confusing aspect of Part A for many, both at the time it was first enacted and currently, is the deductible amount for Part A. The original Medicare Part A deductible was $40 a year for inpatient hospital services. Medicare in 1965 covered 60 days of inpatient services during any particular spell or episode of illness. The deductible was scheduled to rise over time to reflect increases in the average cost of a hospital day. After these 60 days, Medicare covered 30 days of hospitalization with a daily coinsurance rate set at 25 percent of the deductible. It also covered posthospital extended care (such as a nursing home) for up to 100 days and up to 100 posthospital home health visits. Outpatient diagnostic services were covered with a 20 percent coinsurance rates, and there was a lifetime

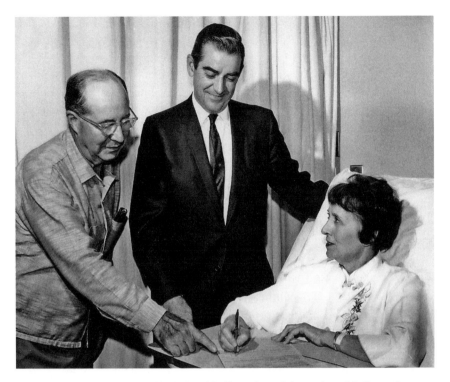

Lillian Grace Avery, the nation's first Medicare beneficiary, signs Medicare forms at Edward Hospital in Naperville, Illinois, on July 1, 1966. (AP Photo)

maximum of 190 days of inpatient psychiatric coverage. In comparison, Medicare now has a $1,068 dollar deductible payment and no copayment for the first 60 days of hospital coverage, a copayment of $267 dollars a day for days 61–90 of hospital coverage, and $534 per "lifetime reserve day" after day 90 of each benefit period (up to 60 days over a lifetime). All costs must be paid for each day after the lifetime reserve days. Inpatient mental health care in a psychiatric hospital is still limited to 190 days in a lifetime.

Part B is the supplementary health insurance portion, sometimes known as SMI or supplementary medial insurance. This provides coverage for physician services, home health services, and a variety of other outpatient services. The financing for Part B of Medicare does not relate to a payroll tax, nor does it have a current working generation helping to cover the costs of current recipients as does the Part A payroll tax. Part B is financed by a combination of monthly premiums levied on current beneficiaries and federal general revenues (tax dollars). The premium is $96.40 per month for most people at present, although the premium can now be higher if the income of the person or couple is high enough (those people will be charged more). This premium change is one of those basic assumptions of the Medicare program as described at the beginning of the chapter. In 1965, when

Medicare began, the premium was three dollars a month. Many who are covered by Medicare do not realize they pay a premium, because generally the premium is deducted from a person's Social Security payment. When people receive their Social Security payment, many do not pay attention to the amount deducted for Medicare. In 1965, Part B covered payment for 80 percent of "reasonable charges" for physician services for office visits, surgery, and consultation, after a $50 deductible. Home health services were covered for up to 100 days a year with a coinsurance of 20 percent. Outpatient psychiatric and mental health treatment required a 50 percent copayment. Diagnostic laboratory tests, x-ray tests, and ambulance services were also covered. The deductible amount in 2009 is $135. Medicare still covers 80 percent of reasonable charges for office visits, surgery, and consultations, meaning that a 20 percent coinsurance is required.

Parts C and D of Medicare

Today, there are two additional parts of Medicare: Part C, previously the Medicare + Choice, and now known as the Medicare Advantage Program, and Part D, the Drug Coverage benefit. Medicare Advantage was established in 1997 under the Balanced Budget Act of that year. It was created to provide greater choices and to encourage the elderly to enroll in private plans such as health maintenance organizations (HMOs) and was an expansion and modification of changes enacted in the early 1980s. More details about this option under Medicare will be covered in Section II of this book. In 2004, Part D, or the drug coverage option of Medicare was passed. This was created to provide drug coverage to Medicare recipients, but in a complicated way, as there are a variety of different plans and the specific plans vary from one state to the next. These plans are provided by private health insurance groups, rather than organized as one large federal plan, as were Parts A and B. More details and issues about this option under Medicare will also be covered in Section II of this book.

There was a year between the passage of the Medicare legislation and its early phase of implementation which began July 1, 1966. That preliminary year was very busy, both in public activities and behind-the-scenes activities. There were major tasks of informing the American public, especially those ages 65 and over, to make sure that they understood the new program and their rights to coverage and benefits. One of the more challenging aspects of this public education was to inform people that they needed to actually enroll in the Part B portion of Medicare in order to have their three-dollar monthly payment withheld from their Social Security check. The Social Security Administration began a large public service campaign, using both national and local media sources to inform the public, especially the elderly, of the new program. In addition, the elderly who were on public assistance needed to be informed of the slightly different ways in which they would participate in the program. Over half of the states took responsibility for informing this group of the details of the new program as it would apply to them. While these were massive tasks, they were generally completed successfully. By the end of the first year of the operation of Medicare, 93 percent of the elderly (about 19 million people at that time in the United States) had enrolled in the Part B program. Beyond enrollment, usage of the program rapidly grew. By the end of the first year of operation, one in five of the elderly had entered a hospital using their Medicare benefits and 12 million of the elderly had used their Part B services. On average, about 80 percent of the hospital expenses of the group using hospital services were paid that year by Medicare (Marmor, 2000).

Less visible to the public, but just as important as informing people about the new program, was the task of evaluating health care facilities whose bills would be paid by Medicare (hospitals, nursing homes, and home health agencies). The law required that facilities which agreed to participate in the new program had to meet specific conditions, including those relating to standards of care and proof that their services were provided on a nondiscriminatory basis in compliance with the Civil Rights Act of 1964. This latter requirement was especially difficult to meet in some portions of the South, and, in reality, there were southern hospitals that did not completely meet this requirement but received program payments during the first year of operation. Operationally, this manipulation of the rules was allowed because one of the early concerns was to be sure that Medicare benefits were not denied to those in formerly segregated areas of the southern United States.

There were some, perhaps not unexpected, problems during the implementation of this new and large government program. Delays occurred in the payment of providers, especially during the first summer of operation. Fears about the possible overcrowding of hospitals, however, did not occur. While some physicians did not cooperate with the program, the cooperation of physicians was high overall. The President of the American Medical Association at the time, James Appel, was helpful in urging physicians to cooperate (at one time there had been talk of a physician boycott) and the organization provided consultations about how to participate, leading to high rates of utilization from physicians. There is a certain irony about the ways that Medicare benefitted physicians after its passage. Physicians, through the efforts of the American Medical Association, were among the most hostile critics of Medicare prior to its passage, and argued that it would destroy the strength and operation of physician services in the United States. Actually, physicians initially received substantial income supplements from the Medicare program and most ended up being reimbursed for services they often previously provided free, or at a reduced cost to the elderly. At the time of the passage of Medicare, most experts agreed that it would help with hospital funding through the improved capacity of elderly patients to pay their hospital bills, and it would also help insurance companies who no longer would be pressured to provide affordable health insurance to the elderly, a group whose medical costs was considered by insurers to be too difficult to predict. An improvement in physicians' abilities to collect their fees did not receive much discussion or attention prior to the passage of Medicare, but it became a reality in the early years of the program.

COSTS OF MEDICARE AND UTILIZATION IN THE EARLY YEARS

Much of what occurred in the first decade of the operation of Medicare was partially expected, but both the total amount of utilization and the costs became issues. In the early years, Medicare costs exceeded the actuarial projections that were made at the time of the passage of the program. One explanation is that both hospital and doctor fees rose, partially because the arrangements for paying physicians were quite generous. There are estimates that physician fees initially rose 5 to 8 percent and physician incomes went up 11 percent (Marmor, 2000). The entire method used to pay both physicians and hospitals was also an issue for Medicare. There was no specific limit set in the statutes passing Medicare that determined what a doctor could charge the patient. Instead, doctors were allowed to be paid "reasonable" charges. A definition provided for reasonable charges was one customary for the individual physician, and no higher than charges in the area or regularly paid by Medicare's program administrators, usually Blue Cross for hospital expenses and Blue Shield for Part B physician expenses. There was an expectation that physicians would charge more than they had previously collected from some poor, elderly patients, since Medicare was not considered to be a charity program and there was a concern that Medicare patients should not be treated as charity cases. As the first year was underway, however, it became clear that there was no agreement either among physicians, or within the government about what the upper limit should be for prevailing medical fees. There was not much preexisting knowledge available about what physicians were actually charging patients. Medicare began with an open-ended method of paying physicians, and concerns grew among physicians that there would be codification and freezing of their fees by the fiscal intermediaries. In a related way, concerns also grew among government officials that costs would be much higher than initial estimates.

Similar problems, perhaps of a more serious nature, existed in the area of establishing hospital costs. The Labor Department's consumer price survey showed that the average daily service charge in American hospitals increased 21.9 percent in the first year of operation of Medicare. By the summer of 1967, it was clear to the Johnson administration that this could grow to be a very big financial problem, and John Gardner, the Secretary of the Department of Health, Education, and Welfare, was given the task of studying the reasons behind the large service charge increase. The eventual report noted that by requiring hospitals to initially reexamine their costs and charges, many had increased their charges (West, 1971). Although hospital costs continued to increase in the second year of the program, the rate of increase was not as large. Other factors, however, continued to push increases in hospital costs. Allowances for depreciation and capital costs were taken into account in the determination of hospital reimbursement rates, and this created a built-inflation push. In 1968 and 1969, Medicare costs rose around 40 percent each year, thus acquiring a reputation both in Congress and in the administrative branch as a program with a potential to be an uncontrollable burden on the federal budget.

One clear result of the first two years of Medicare's existence was that the rise in medical costs initially lead to increased interest in national health insurance. For example, in 1968, a Committee for National Health Insurance was created by organized labor and the American Hospital Association announced that it planned to study the feasibility of a national health insurance plan. Some of these initiatives were related to the experience of certain states with the Medicaid program for the poor which emerged at the same time as Medicare. In the large states of New York and California, the Medicaid program brought about great financial pressures, as a much higher than predicted utilization together with price increases added to the initial cost of the program, both to the states and to the federal government.

Medicare proved to be a more complex program to administer and to control costs than the Social Security program. For the latter program, most administrative issues were internal and pension expenditures for Social Security were quite predictable and based upon clear formulas. In contrast, Medicare costs were varied and based upon how much the elderly used care, how much doctors and hospitals charged for this care, and by changes in medical technology that made new procedures available. These three factors led to additional costs and made it difficult to predict the rising costs for Medicare. Moreover, the administration of many aspects of these costs was not controlled by the government, but by the fiscal intermediaries. While these groups provided a buffer between the Social Security administration and doctors and hospitals, they also weakened government control and had a long history of intimate relationships with providers. The lack of clear definitions of terms and procedures left open the possibility that providers could increase their revenue in ways that the government had not anticipated. The Social Security administrators, who were not yet that experienced with working with their counterparts in health care, had not anticipated these issues. The initial emphasis of the administrators was to cooperate with providers and get them to participate and have a smooth beginning to Medicare, as they had in the 1930s with Social Security.

In hindsight, it is easy to criticize some of these early decisions, but when Medicare was first enacted, the mandate was to provide services to the elderly without significantly interfering with the traditional organization of American medicine.

While issues of the administration of Medicare became more distinct, and a concern about costs became more common, the issues of controlling costs were not as easy. While the rate of hospital costs did decrease from the 20 percent of the first year, over the next five years of the program, the rate averaged 14 percent (West, 1971). Similarly, while the rate of growth in physician fees was the highest in 1966 (7.8%), the rate over the next five years remained quite high, at 6.8 percent. This rate of growth in Medicare costs meant that by 1970 there was agreement between administrators within the federal government, and between both Republican and Democratic politicians, that the increasing costs of medical care were becoming a crisis. One reaction was to focus on overall reform of the health care system, not just on changes in the Medicare program while a different reaction was to focus on changes and initiatives within the program.

A key issue in Medicare policy became the discussion of different ways to control costs through regulatory approaches and financing reforms. This was especially true in Congress, since the primary legislative location for the oversight of the Medicare program was the House Committee on Ways and Means and the Senate Finance Committee. Traditionally, these congressional committees have focused on norms of financial responsibility. In 1972, the Social Security Amendments of that year established professional standards review organizations (PSROs). These organizations were to review the care received by federally funded patients as well as to encourage the development of HMOs and the enrollment of Medicare recipients in them, review capital spending of hospitals and allow for federal support for state experiments with prospective payment systems. In 1974, the Health Planning and Resource Development Act, Public Law 93641, created over 200 health systems agencies to oversee medical planning and resources use. As various political issues shifted in the 1970s, no major national health insurance reform was passed and the partial planning-based reforms were eventually judged to be ineffective, became sources of political concern, and were eventually dismantled. With the benefit of hindsight, most policy analysts now agree that these partial reforms were inadequate measures for controlling rising health care costs and did little to impact the basic inflationary structure of medical care in the United States. Actually, only a few changes in Medicare coverage and benefits occurred in the early years of the program. In 1967, a 60-day reserve for hospitalization along with a 50 percent coinsurance rate was added. More of the changes enacted in the 1970s are discussed in the next section of this chapter.

One other issue that became clear in the first few years of Medicare was that while the program greatly improved the health care access of the elderly, it did not solve all of their problems in terms of access to care. (This was also the one reason contributing to the continued discussion of some form of national health insurance.) Medicare had various limitations on coverage, and beneficiaries were responsible for considerable amounts of deductibles and coinsurance, both for Part A, hospital costs and for Part B, physician costs. Also, Medicare did not provide coverage for what we now call "long-term care," although at the time the higher costs of chronic illness were under discussion. Home health and nursing home services were mostly restricted to short-term stays, immediately following a hospital visit. This was comparable to many private insurance packages, but it was much less than had initially been proposed as part of Truman's national health insurance provisions. It was also less than what some of the poor elderly had received under Kerr-Mills, the joint federal-state health insurance program for low-income elderly that had been enacted in 1960. Those provisions later became part of Medicaid, and eventually became one of the ways in which the Medicaid program in most states now pays as much in long-term care for the poor elderly as it does for care of poor children and their mothers, the groups thought of as the main recipients of the Medicaid program when it was passed.

CHANGES IN MEDICARE FROM 1972 TO 1980

The changes in the Medicare program from 1972 to 1980 tended to either fall into the categories of expansion (such as expanding eligibility and areas of coverage for those already eligible for the program), and continued attempts to deal with rising costs and with the administration of the program. In the area of expansion, some important additional services for Medicare occurred during this time period for people already eligible. In 1972, some chiropractic services, speech therapy, and physical therapy were added as benefits to those who already qualified for Medicare. One of the largest expansions in that year was the extension of Medicare services to people who required hemodialysis or renal transplants for kidney problems by declaring them disabled. While this expansion represented a numerically small category, the average medical expenses for these individuals were quite high, making the coverage very important to them. Also, many experts thought this expansion would allow national health insurance coverage for more people, as it represented the first specific disease category to be covered, although including specific disease groups had not been part of the early discussions of Medicare. Although the expectation was that additional disease categories might be added to the Medicare program in the future, this expectation was not met. The National Kidney Foundation and physician kidney specialists were important groups that lobbied for the inclusion of patients needing hemodialysis, a very expensive procedure, under Medicare. As the high costs of this new disease category became more evident, costs alone became a reason for less expansion into other disease categories.

In addition, Medicare coverage was extended to Social Security beneficiaries on disability insurance. Including the disabled in Medicare had been recommended by the 1965 Advisory Council on Social Security and was proposed by the Johnson administration in 1967. This expansion had been actually passed by both the House and the Senate in 1970, but it was not enacted and instead, was held up as part of broader negotiations over Medicare legislation that year in a conference committee. Taken together, these provisions broadened the reach of Medicare beyond the elderly to include substantial numbers of people less than 65 years of age. Fifteen years after the passage of this expansion, there were three million nonelderly recipients of Medicare, including about 100,000 dialysis patients. All together, these figures represented 10 percent of all program enrollees, a clear demonstration of how what may seem to be small, specialized expansions can become important (and also expensive) parts of Medicare (West, 1971).

There might have been expectations of continued additions to Medicare benefits, but during this time period, only a few additional services were added to the program. In 1980, more home health benefits were added by eliminating the limit on the number of home health visits, the prior hospitalization requirement, and the deductible for any Part B benefits. Also in 1980, the amendments began an exploration of inclusion of surgical procedures that could be done on an outpatient basis in an ambulatory surgical center. In these cases, reimbursement would be based upon a prospective payment system. However, the expansion of benefits in Medicare did not match the expansion of benefits in the typical private health insurance plan. By 1980, people with good health insurance coverage often had dental care insurance (about 50 percent of private plans) and drug coverage (about 25 percent of private plans), both of which were not added to Medicare. Broader, large expansions generally did not occur, partially due to fiscal concerns about the program. Other explanations for lack of greater expansions are the development of private supplemental insurance, and confusion of beneficiaries about Medicare coverage (Oberlander, 2003).

Fiscal concerns about Medicare continued to grow during the 1970s. The dialysis benefits added in 1972 quickly experienced cost overruns, adding to the image of fiscal recklessness that Medicare was acquiring among some members of Congress. The fiscal concerns are one explanation for why an expansionary agenda for Medicare did not occur. Given the fiscal pressures with the administrative agency, and given the awareness among policy experts, interest groups for the elderly that might have pushed expansion recognized that the political environment was becoming hostile to Medicare expansion. For some of the interest groups for the elderly, their focus became the protection of existing benefits and existing beneficiary groups rather than expanding benefits or groups.

In addition to changes in benefits, some changes in the administration of Medicare occurred in this time period. In 1977, one of the amendments passed reorganized the administration of the Medicare program from that of the Social Security Administration. In the 1977 amendments, the Health Care Financing Administration (later renamed the Centers for Medicare and Medicaid Services) was created. HCFA, as the new agency quickly became known, became responsible for the administration of both Medicare and Medicaid. This change was part of a broader reorganization of the Department of Health, Education, and Welfare that moved education into a different agency. Combining both Medicare and Medicaid together into an agency that focused on issues of health financing was seen as one way to achieve administrative cost savings. This move to combine the administration of the two programs was one factor in the transformation of Medicare from a social insurance program to a health financing program and eventually, weakened the ties between Social Security and Medicare. One way to think about this change is a shift from an emphasis on claims payment to protect beneficiaries to a focus on cost containment as a primary administrative task.

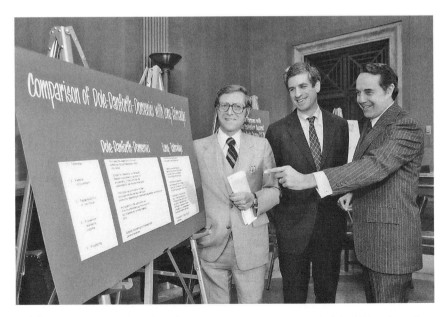

Three Republican senators are pictured in Washington, March 26, 1979, where they announced their intention to introduce "The Catastrophic Health Insurance and Medicare Amendments of 1979." Standing with charts which compare their proposal to another slated for introduction are, from left: Pete Domenici, New Mexico; John Danforth, Missouri; and Bob Dole, Kansas. (AP Photo/Harrity)

The last major change in the 1980 amendments to Medicare was the provision of oversight and coordination to Medicare supplemental insurance, also called "Medigap," and the establishment of a voluntary certification program for Medigap policies. These were important changes, since the establishment of supplemental health insurance for the aged has helped to create a source of stability in Medicare benefits (Oberlander, 2003). Medigap supplemental insurance policies help provide beneficiaries with insurance to cover gaps in services and cost sharing required by Medicare. While not anticipated as important at the time of creation of Medicare, these supplemental policies have answered the desires of beneficiaries to have all, or almost all, of their costs covered by a routine payment (such as the monthly Part B payment and a supplemental Medigap monthly payment).

Many retirees prefer to know in advance what their medical costs will be each month, whether or not they have major health problems, so that their expenses are more predictable. Given the limited scope of Medicare benefits, this desire on the part of consumers created a market niche for private insurance which moved to provide this type of policy. Almost from the beginning of Medicare, the desire of beneficiaries to have more thorough coverage was indicated, and in 1967, 46 percent of elderly Medicare beneficiaries had some form of private supplemental insurance (Cafferata, 1985; Rice, 1987). By 1984, that figure had increased to 72 percent, and the Baucus amendments of 1980 were designed to help clarify the various Medigap policies so that elderly consumers would have a better understanding of what they were purchasing and what would be covered.

In general, supplemental plans pay for cost-sharing expenses for Medicare-covered services. Almost all plans cover the deductible and coinsurance portions for Part A hospital care, and most cover the 20 percent copayment for Part B physician services. Prior to the enactment of the drug plan or Part D of Medicare, less than half of Medigap policies covered prescription drugs. Also, less than half covered the physician bill portion that was in excess of what Medicare covered as "reasonable" charges. Plans also varied on whether they covered additional hospital days. Some services were rarely covered, such as additional nursing home days, coverage of nursing home stays not certified by Medicare, dental care, eyeglasses, or hearing aids.

Most Medicare beneficiaries received supplemental coverage either as a benefit of current or previous employment or individually purchased a Medigap plan. In the mid-1980s, about a third of the elderly had this coverage as a benefit of past or current employment, with the employer paying most of the costs, while the rest purchased it as supplemental coverage from private insurance companies. Politically, these supplemental policies, however paid for, had an important political impact on the Medicare program, by holding down pressures for expansion of benefits. This is similar to the role private insurance now plays in some countries with public health insurance, where extras such as dental care and eye care or a private room in a hospital may be provided by supplemental insurance. Not surprisingly, certain population groups are more likely to carry Medigap policies. Income, race, education status, and health status all impact the likelihood of having Medigap coverage. Whites and those with higher education are much more likely to have coverage, as are those with incomes double the poverty level. Of course, those with low enough incomes have Medicaid as dually eligible beneficiaries to pick up the copayments and deductibles of Medicare. Those individuals in better health are more likely to have coverage than those in poor health, which may seem unusual, but is probably linked to the latter also having lower incomes and education (Rice and McCall, 1985; Garfinkel et al., 1987). Thus, individuals who are most likely to need the supplemental coverage due to poor health are less likely to actually have the coverage.

There is also a connection to the political realities of the Medicare program. We know that political activism in the United States is linked with socioeconomic status, with those of higher social position being more politically active. Given the linkage of Medigap policies with social factors, the most politically active of the elderly have less personally based interest in agitating for greater benefits. The new provisions passed in 1980 recognized how popular supplemental policies were becoming, and provided a way for the government to make sure that people spent their supplemental funds wisely and understood what the different plans would cover by requiring more uniform types of policies and information about policies.

By the beginning of the 1980s, Medicare had become a critical program for the elderly and disabled. It was an imperfect program, which did not cover all the health care costs of these groups. Moreover, concerns about the costs of the program were becoming larger issues in Congress, at the same time that concerns of beneficiaries about better coverage were being discussed. Changes from the early days to 1980 dealt with a limited range of problems. Because Medicare is always subject to changes by Congress, new issues arise every few years and new solutions and ideas are covered. Some of the most important changes occurred from 1980 to 2000 and will be discussed in the next chapter of this section.

CHAPTER 3

Changes in Medicare from the 1980s to the 1990s: A Focus on Types of Cost Reforms

This chapter will review some of the major Medicare changes that were enacted (and in one case, then cancelled the next year) from 1980 to 2000. The chapter will also point out some of the consistencies in the Medicare program during this time period. Changes from 2000 and later will be covered as part of the discussion of current themes in Medicare in Section II of this book with one exception. The one exception is that issues related to Medicare and managed care will be discussed in Section II of the book, rather than in this chapter of Section I, even though some of the changes made as part of the implementation of Medicare managed-care programs (also known as the Medicare Choice Plan) were also enacted from the 1980s to the 1990s.

While not all of the major changes to Medicare in this time period were financial- or payment-based, two of the most important were modifications as to how hospitals were paid under Medicare and modifications as to how physicians were paid through Medicare. By 1980, Medicare had become the second largest domestic program, as well as the fastest growing program, making a focus on costs likely (Moon, 1993). Both the costs of health care overall, and of Medicare more specifically, were steadily increasing by 1980. The proportion of the U.S. gross national product (GNP) spent on medical care increased from 7.1 percent in 1970 to 8.9 percent in 1980 (Moon, 1993). While not all of this increased spending was due to rising Medicare costs, they contributed to the larger problem of annual increases in overall health spending. Other Chapter 3 topics to be covered include the issue of trust funds, especially as linked to financing and funding during this period, and issues of benefits' stability, the role of supplemental health insurance plans, and the controversy about the Medicare Catastrophic Coverage Act.

TEFRA, DRG REFORMS, AND CHANGES IN THE 1980S

The Reagan administration supported major changes in the Medicare program during this time period. The majority of the enacted changes, as well as some proposed changes that were not enacted, were attempts to deal with the problem of rising health care costs. However, there were some changes to Medicare that added to the costs, despite the growing concerns. One such change, from the 1982 Medicare Hospice Benefit legislation, was the coverage of hospice services. While there were (and are) reasons for arguing that, in the long run, covering hospice services may decrease end-of-life costs as well as improve the end of life for dying people, this change was less related to cost concerns than to quality concerns. The hospice movement provided (and continues to provide) an important service for the elderly. The Medicare Hospice Benefit in 1982 spurred the rapid growth of hospice programs across the United States. To qualify for hospice care, patients were required to have a life expectancy of six months or less, as determined by their attending physician. Patients also signed an agreement which acknowledged their terminal condition and waived their traditional Medicare coverage (which paid for curative medical care) in favor of the palliative care (non-curative) offered by hospice. The Medicare Hospice Benefit reimbursed hospices by means of a standard per diem rate of payment per patient, which was presumed to cover the costs of all goods and services provided to patients.

Another major change in the 1982 Tax Equity and Fiscal Responsibility Act (TEFRA) increased the Part B premium to cover 25 percent of program costs. This was part of a group of policies, as with some others that had already been enacted in 1981, that were designed to slow the growth of Medicare spending by bringing in more revenue from covered recipients. TEFRA also required federal employees to begin paying the health insurance payroll tax. The end result of this change was to make almost all federal civilian employees in the United States covered by Medicare by the time they retired. The Act also expanded the Health Care Financing Administration's (later renamed the Centers for Medicare and Medicaid Services) quality oversight efforts by replacing professional standards review organizations (PSROs) with peer review organizations (PROs). TEFRA also imposed a ceiling on the amount Medicare would pay for a hospital discharge.

These 1982 changes to Medicare were of a limited nature, as contrasted with a major change in reimbursement policies for Medicare that was enacted in 1983. In that year, Congress created the Medicare prospective payment system, which based payments to hospitals on predetermined rates per discharges from hospitals for diagnosis-related groups (DRGs). This system replaced the way hospitals had been paid since the implementation of Medicare. That older system was still being used by most large health insurance companies in the United States to reimburse hospitals for care, so the DRG system for Medicare was a major change in hospital payment approaches. The earlier approach used a cost-based system of reimbursement in which hospitals provided Medicare with their costs for each part of the hospital visit—the per day per room charge, the charges for special services used such as a hospital operating room or diagnostic technology, and the cost of supplies used in the care of the patient. The DRG system was a major departure from how payment had occurred in the past, and was the creation of a complex system that was regulatory in content. However, before the system could be implemented, the federal government had to provide detailed regulations that explained how the new system would work. The new legislation forced hospitals that received Medicare funds (basically all U.S. hospitals) to reorganize how they were paid for Medicare patients.

This was an interesting policy change at the time, since the Reagan administration was philosophically committed to competition and the private marketplace as the determinants of the distribution of health care resources. This highly regulated approach seemed not to fit well with the overall philosophy of the Reagan administration. Rising health care costs were viewed as a greater threat to planned tax cuts and other policy goals of the administration than the enactment of a reimbursement policy that was regulatory in nature and wholly at odds with the Reagan administration approach to policy. If rising Medicare costs threatened the rest of the Reagan administration plans, then a regulatory strategy to hold down health costs in Medicare was acceptable. This payment change, along with the payment change for physicians discussed in the next section, have been described by some health policy experts as the most significant developments in Medicare policy since its inception (Marmor, 2000).

The DRG change resulted in converting Medicare payments to hospitals to a prospective per case system based on the diagnosis of the patient which included more than 460 different diagnostic-related payment categories. The model was based on a program in New Jersey that had experimented with DRGs as a way to pay hospitals. It was adopted by the Reagan administration as a way to hold down rising hospital costs. Under the new system, instead of a hospital charging Medicare a set fee per day plus specific charges for supplies and other facilities used in the care of a patient, the hospital care of a Medicare patient was paid with one fee set in advance, based upon the expected average length of stay and the services typically used for that diagnosis. A hospital's payment for its operating costs is calculated using a national standardized amount, which is higher for hospitals located in urban areas. The amount is adjusted by the use of wage indexes associated with the area in which the hospital is located. (This is in addition to the use of the DRG for the specific patient based on the diagnosis.) Additional payments can be made for cases with extraordinary costs (known as outliers), costs linked to a hospital participating in graduate medical education, and for hospitals that serve a disproportionate share of low-income patients. In a short period of time, Medicaid also started to reimburse hospitals in most states using the DRG system and many private insurance companies soon followed.

This Medicare change then led to major reform in hospital payment approaches across the United States for a variety of payers of health care to try and force hospitals to provide care more economically. Under the older retrospective payment approach, hospitals could be almost certain of breaking even or having excess revenues on the care of every patient, except for charity cases or bad debts (which no one paid). Now, hospitals had to figure out how to provide care in such a way that they still broke even on the care of Medicare patients (and later, many others). Because people over the age of 65 use hospital care services at a much higher rate than younger age groups, initially this change impacted half or more of all hospital stays. One concern was that hospitals would shift costs to privately financed patients, thus having a positive impact on Medicare costs but not on overall medical inflation. A related concern was that hospitals would become reluctant to take Medicare patients and prefer patients with more lucrative reimbursements. Given the importance of Medicare patients to hospitals in terms of numbers, this did not become a problem. In essence, this Medicare policy change provided a common set of operating procedures and included detailed regulations to ensure that care for Medicare patients did not suffer as a result of payment reforms.

What was the impact of these changes in Medicare reimbursement for hospitals on overall hospital and Medicare costs? The general consensus is that the DRG hospital payment reform did help to contain the growth in hospital costs at least initially and to some extent. Admission rates to hospitals declined from 1983 through 1987, and rates in 1989 for people ages 65 and over were still only 85 percent of the rates in 1983 (Christensen, 1991). The rate of growth in annual hospital expenses slowed for a few years after the implementation of the DRG system, although the rate of growth began again to increase later. From 1985 to 1990, hospital expenditures under Medicare declined from 28.9 percent of total national hospital expenditures to 26.1 percent (Letsch et al., 1992). Similarly, Medicare's per capita expenditures initially grew less rapidly than the per capita expenditures of people with private health insurance.

Some early fears about the system implementation were that hospitals would discharge sick patients too quickly, leading to unnecessary hospital readmissions. There was even some evidence that this occurred during the early phases of the DRG payment system (Gay et al., 1989). Soon, reforms in payment of readmissions were put into place, so that readmissions within a too short period of time no longer generated the start of a new DRG payment for that hospitalization. Length of stay dropped by about 0.9 days in 1984 and 0.6 days in 1985, compared to an average drop of 0.2 days per year from 1967 to 1983 (Koch, 1988). For the majority of patients, it no longer seemed that access to medical care has decreased under DRG reimbursement (DesHarnais et al., 1987).

In 1984, the Deficit Reduction Act (DEFRA) was passed as a way to address rising health care costs through changes in payments to both hospitals and physicians. This legislation placed a limit upon the rate of increases in the DRG payments that would be allowed in the two years following the DEFRA legislation. In 1985, the Graham-Rudman-Hollins Act established mandatory deficit reduction targets for a longer period of time—the following five years. This resulted in some impact upon the Medicare program, leading to cuts in payments to both hospitals and physicians. Other smaller changes also occurred such as an adjustment in payments to hospitals that served a disproportionate share of poor patients, resulting in higher payments for most of those hospitals. Prospective payment rates were frozen at 1985 levels for part of the next year as a way to hold down health care costs. Payments to hospitals for the indirect costs of medical education were also modified. Payment amounts for capital related costs were reduced under the Omnibus Budget Reconciliation Act of 1987 (OBRA 87) legislation, by 3.5 percent in fiscal year 1987, 7 percent in fiscal year 1988, and 10 percent in fiscal year 1990 (Chapen and Silloway, 1992). Also, some technical adjustments occurred in how DRG payments were calculated for outlier (or extremely expensive) cases.

Tinkering by Congress and by administrative staff that had oversight responsibility for Medicare with other technical aspects, such as the wage index used to calculate hospital payments and capital-related cost formulas, continued (Letsch et al., 1992). Generally, PPS payment rates now are updated annually. There are five types of specialty hospitals that are exempted from PPS reimbursement: psychiatric, rehabilitation, long-term care, children's, and cancer hospitals. As this brief explanation of some of the aspects and changes in Medicare reimbursement makes clear, the technical rules and their changes become quite complex, and it is not possible to explain every change or the details of exact aspects of reimbursement. In most years, there are new specific changes in payment issues, but these become too detailed to cover every change, and each change is not important enough to review in detail. While some books do provide details on reimbursement policies (O'Sullivan et al., 2003), new legislation and regulations can cause the material to quickly become outdated.

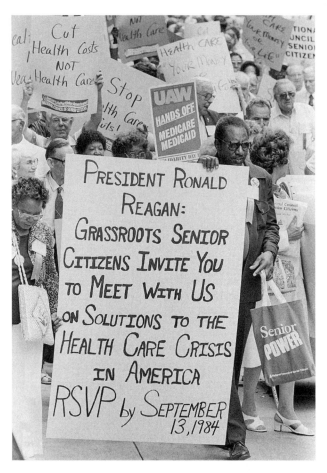

Members of the National Council of Senior Citizens carry signs protesting what they called President Ronald Reagan's health care cuts during a protest march on June 28, 1984 in downtown Philadelphia. (AP Photo/George Widman)

Due to the impact of changes to the DRG payment approach as well as other changes that impacted overall use of hospital care, it is now clear that hospitals have shifted more care into outpatient settings. One reason is to maximize revenues, since the DRG payment system applies only to inpatient care; hospitals can maximize revenues by increasing outpatient admissions. A survey of physicians found general agreement that, under PPS (Prospective Payment Systems), hospitals have encouraged more outpatient testing (Guterman and Dobson, 1986). One summary of the impact of the DRG approach argued that while inpatient hospital care use declined initially and then stabilized from 1987 onwards, outpatient hospital costs continued to increase, as did costs for physician care (Edwards and Fischer, 1989). This means that the actual impact of the DRG payment reform system has been less than hoped for initially. As often happens in health care with a reform that impacts only one payer and only one type of service, hospitals and other providers learn to "game" the system. That is, providers maximize revenue given the new rules, in this case by shifting some care to the outpatient setting that has not had the same payment reform. This is one of the reasons that healthcare analysts often argue that piecemeal reforms of the health care system generally lead to overall disappointing results.

The prospective payment approach to reimbursement of facilities was extended beyond hospitals by the Balanced Budget Act of 1997. This legislation established a prospective payment system for home health agencies and for skilled nursing facilities. It also limited or eliminated payments in a number of other areas. Health care provider groups were quite concerned about these changes and cuts, and argued that some facilities would be forced to close and limit access to services to people on Medicare. In November 1999, Congress passed funding increases to mitigate the impact of the 1997 provisions.

PHYSICIAN REFORM AND RBRVS

The DRG system change was a major reform to the way hospitals were paid which covered one large part of Medicare costs. Another large part of Medicare costs are fees paid to physicians. It made sense then, as attempts to control costs and to have payments linked to what are seen as positive outcomes for Medicare, that the next area of major payment reform involved physician fees. There had been continuing and substantial increases in Medicare Part B (physician) expenditures. Throughout the 1980s, a variety of smaller, incremental measures to try and control physician costs had been implemented. These included the 1984 Deficit Reduction Act (DEFRA) which temporarily (for two-and-a-half-years) froze increases in physician payment under Medicare. Despite this legislation, Medicare's physician expenditures continued to increase. In fact, the implementation and initial success of the DRG hospital-payment reform meant that after that system was put into place, Medicare physician expenditures increased at a rate three times that for hospital payments (Epstein and Blumenthal, 1993). At the same time, there was a mandate that the Office of Technology Assessment study alternative ways to pay physicians which would serve as a guide for physician-payment Medicare reform. The same Act also created a differential between two classes of physicians under Medicare: participating and nonparticipating.

As another interim move, the Omnibus Budget Reconciliation Act of 1987 (OBRA 87) reduced physician fees for 12 procedures that experts concluded were being paid at too high a rate, and also provided higher fee increases for primary care rather than for specialty care. In 1986, the Physician Payment Review Commission (PPRC) was created by Congress to help in developing a fee schedule to be used to pay physicians and to aid in health policymaking. This followed the approach used with hospital reimbursement with the creation of a special group, the Prospective Payment Assessment Commission (ProPAC), to monitor the implementation of hospital payment reform.

Major physician payment reform was part of the Omnibus Budget Reconciliation Act of 1989 (OBRA 89) legislation. Congress directed the Health Care Financing Administration (HCFA), the agency in charge of Medicare at that time, to begin implementing a resource-based relative value scale (RBRVS) as the way to pay physicians for services delivered to Medicare recipients. The system began in January 1992 and was not without controversy. Physician groups launched protests in June of that year when the draft regulations were initially released. The American Medical Association (AMA) was so concerned that they threatened to seek Congressional action to challenge the proposed new reimbursement system (McIlrath, 1991a).

The RBRVS system is, as with the DRG system, a technical reform that is complex and not easy to explain. The system was initially developed by William Hsiao (Hsiao et al., 1988) who was commissioned by the Health Care Financing Administration (HCFA), the agency responsible for the administration of the Medicare (and the Medicaid) program. Until that point, most physicians and all Medicare physicians were reimbursed based on what they charged for an office visit and for other specific services. The goal of the new Hsiao system was to determine how long it takes physicians to perform various kinds of tasks. Each service a physician might provide was assigned a relative weight based upon three geographically adjusted values for work, practice costs, and malpractice insurance premiums. Then, a new payment approach was created, relative to the time and resources used for each task. The goal was to develop a system to pay physicians based on objective measures of complexity, time, and resources involved in the delivery of physician services. In the final application of this approach, a scale of relative weightings or relative values was formed as the basis of the new physician reimbursement system (Hsaio et al., 1988). The assumption of federal policymakers was that recalculating physician payments based on "objective" measures of relative value would end up with smaller payments for specialized medical care providers such as surgeons and somewhat higher payments for primary care physicians. The hope was that the new system, through reducing the "value" of specialized services, would reduce physician expenditures because of a system of financial incentives that favored the less expensive primary care.

Given the complaints directed at the initial drafts, some of the rules were revised by Health Care Financing Administration (HCFA). The initial rules would have slightly increased the fees paid to generalist physicians and decreased fees paid to specialists. After negotiations with groups from organized medicine (such as the AMA), changes were adopted with others implemented along the way. These occurred gradually from 1992 to 1996. By 1996, payments for family physicians were increased by 30 percent and payments for procedure-oriented specialists were decreased by a similar amount (McIlrath, 1991b). During the initial implementation, it was decided that if the payment for a service was less than 15 percent more than the determined RBRVS rate, then that service was placed immediately under the new RBRVS payment system. If the difference was larger, initial year payments were a blend of the RBRVS approach and the older payment system. The earlier distinction between full participating doctors and others became more important under RBRVS. If the physician agreed to be a full participating doctor and accept the Medicare rate as payment in full for all cases, the physician received a full amount according to the payment schedule. If the physician did not become a participating physician, the physician received only 95 percent of the scheduled amount. Because prior to the new system, rates varied from state to state in relationship to prevailing doctor's rates in that state, the impact on doctors varied from state to state. The December 1991 revised rules increased average payment levels in 16 states and four specialties. This legislation created volume performance standards that would reduce physician payments in future years if certain spending targets were exceeded. There were also new restrictions on how much physicians could bill Medicare beneficiaries in excess of federal reimbursement rates.

As with the adoption of the DRG system by Ronald Reagan, a conservative Republican President, the RBRVS reform was signed into law by President George H. W. Bush, another conservative Republican. The latter reform was enacted with bipartisan political support, low public visibility and discussion, and ultimately, the agreement of the medical industry, despite complaints about specific aspects and regulations related to the new system. As with the DRG system, the RBRVS system was a regulatory reform that, in actuality, was the introduction of an administered pricing system by the federal government enacted by a conservative Republican administration (although generally in American politics conservatives are not in favor of greater government regulation and government-administered pricing systems). One reason for this is that the regulation of medical providers was presented not as a regulatory reform, but as a system backed by science and research that focused on technical proficiency and objectivity. Students of the American political system in general, as well as its application to health care, have argued that while Americans often distrust politics and politicians, and therefore avoid policy solutions that rely on trust from that group, they are more in favor of mechanistic, self-enforcing solutions (Morone, 1990). Initially, the RBRVS physician-payment reform fit this type of solution so it was easier to present to the American public. Over time, despite the technical imagery of the RBRVS program, the result of the new approach was a pattern of strengthened federal authority over medical care providers, as also happened with DRG payment reform for hospitals.

The approach did initially lead to a slowdown in the growth of Medicare payments to physicians. In the five years before the enactment of RBRVS, Part B (physician) expenditures rose at an average annual rate of 10.3 percent. The rise in physician expenditures was not as large in the five years following the enactment of RBRVS, with an increase of 5.6 percent in the five years after RBRVS (Health Care Financing Administration, 1998). Medicare payments also declined as a percentage of private rates, which shows a slowing in the rate of growth in federal payments for physicians. By 1993, Medicare fees for physician services were 62 percent of private sector rates, down from 71 percent in 1989. Thus, the RBRVS system demonstrated some success in slowing Medicare expenditures, and meant that physicians no longer had close-to-total control over their income from Medicare.

Overall, the new fee schedule has some very important limitations. The fee schedule does not affect such factors as the basic incentives built into fee-for-service medicine and the explosion of new medical technologies. Although both physicians and patients want the best and newest medical technologies, these new approaches are most often more expensive than older, less technological approaches. This is one of the factors that lead to rising costs, despite a reformulated way to pay physicians. Nor does the emphasis on rewarding the less procedure-oriented medicine, such as general practice and internal medicine, (by recognizing that it takes time and therefore, will cost money to talk to a patient in more detail) change the overall thrust of the practice of medicine. It is beneficial to recognize that physicians need to take time to talk to patients in order to determine what their current health problems are and what practices and activities of the patient make solving those health problems more difficult. In the long run, physician time is expensive, and holding down physician reimbursement with technical reforms of payment somewhat slows rising costs, but does not really solve cost problems. Moreover, there is a concern that the current determination of relative values, which is updated at various points by a committee of the American Medical Association, the Specialty Society Relative Value Scale Update Committee (RUC), has continued to undervalue many of the services delivered by primary care physicians. Despite the goals when the RBRVS system was first introduced, experts now agree that there is still undervaluing of primary care evaluation and management (E&M) visits and that the system is still too procedure-based.

The failure of the RBRVS reform program to achieve its goals in cost containment and other areas could result in abandonment of fee-for-service compensation of physicians under Medicare, although this has not yet occurred. There are health systems, even within the United States, in which physicians are paid a salary for delivering care and some experts would argue that this approach may be the one that will most restrain rising physician costs. One example of this approach is the Veteran's Administration system of care. Some HMOs such as Kaiser-Permanente also reimburse many of their physicians with this approach and in Great Britain, most hospital-based specialists are paid on a salaried basis. These types of changes, however, might raise major political concerns among Medicare recipients as well as concern among physicians. Many politicians would see such reforms not as technical changes, but as major reforms of the Medicare system. These major reforms have generally been resisted by politicians, the public, and health care providers alike.

STABILITY OF BENEFITS, SUPPLEMENTAL INSURANCE, AND MORE GENERAL FINANCING OF MEDICARE

In the period from 1980 through 2000, as discussed previously in this chapter, one major focus in Medicare was trying to control costs through payment reform, first for hospitals and then for doctors. In his book examining the political life of Medicare, Oberlander (2003) points out that Medicare benefits have been fairly stable, with the first major addition being the passage of prescription drug benefits in 2003, a program that actually began in 2006. This benefit stability is true even though it was not part of one of the basic assumptions of the Medicare program at the time it was first enacted. Oberlander (2003) points out that the architects of the Medicare structure strongly believed that Medicare was just the beginning of the federal government's role in providing health care to a subset of citizens, i.e., the elderly, and that both services and covered groups would expand over time. A well-known political scientist, James Wilson, who wrote about Medicare in 1973, argued that it was a reasonable expectation for benefits to have automatic increases, as was the case with Social Security benefits. Politically, Wilson felt this was likely because Medicare was providing benefits to a large constituency of voters, and program financing was spread broadly across the population, so that legislators could expand benefits and receive political credit for doing so without really creating political "losers."

However, this is not what happened with the Medicare program as benefits did not expand substantially in the decades following the enactment of the program. Why they did not is an interesting issue to pursue. One of the reasons for the enactment of Medicare for the elderly was the popular appeal of this group as especially deserving of governmental help. This view did not change for the first 20 years of the Medicare program. A poll taken in 1986 showed over 80 percent of the public favored, or strongly favored expanding Medicare, including adding nursing home coverage (Cook and Barrett, 1992). In addition, the elderly were widely viewed as a politically powerful group, and special interest groups focused on the

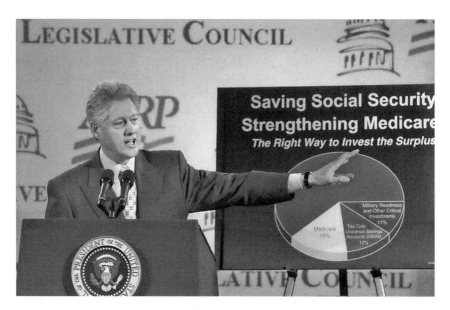

President Bill Clinton pitches his plan to save Social Security and spend the budget surplus during a gathering of the American Association of Retired Persons, AARP, at the Willard Hotel in Washington, D.C., on February 3, 1999. (AP Photo/J. Scott Applewhite)

elderly were growing with the aging of the U.S. population. The American Association for Retired Persons (AARP), the National Committee to Preserve Social Security and Medicare, the National Alliance of Senior Citizens, and the National Council of Senior Citizens were all important lobbying groups for the elderly. The AARP grew from its origins as a group for retired teachers to a general membership group that, by the late 1980s, had become the most visible and influential interest group representing the elderly. Many believed the AARP and other groups would lobby and represent the desires of the elderly and push for expansion of Medicare benefits. Two factors that should have made this easier is that the elderly have a tradition of voting at higher rates than the overall population, and the elderly's share of the voting electorate increased in the years following the passage of Medicare.

Oberlander (2003) argues there are three major reasons why Medicare benefits did not expand as expected: (1) the dominance of fiscal concerns in program policy; (2) the development of private supplemental insurance; and (3) the confusion of beneficiaries over Medicare coverage. The previous two sections of this chapter have demonstrated how fiscal concerns about Medicare ended up becoming paramount issues, and important enough to modify the payment approach to both hospitals and doctors by 1990. Fiscal concerns started early in the program, with Medicare costs being much higher than early actuarial projections. One structural factor within Congress responsible for this concern was that oversight of Medicare was located in the House Committee on Ways and Means and the Senate Finance Committee. As previously mentioned, these are congressional committees that often focus on financial responsibility and attention to finances. This governmental focus on financial restraint led the organizations representing the elderly such as the AARP to emphasize protection of current Medicare benefits rather than an expansion of new benefits.

The second reason for why Medicare did not expand was the creation and growth of supplemental health insurance which became a source of stability for Medicare benefits, and which was not initially expected by the founders of Medicare. Supplemental medical insurance, sometimes called Medigap policies, are private health insurance policies that beneficiaries purchase to cover gaps in Medicare services. Given the desire of many elderly to have first dollar coverage, (that is, not to have to pay copayments each time a health care service is received or to pay deductibles until the limit is reached) many wished to purchase supplemental health insurance to accompany their Medicare benefits. Even in the early years of Medicare, many elderly purchased some type of supplement (almost half in 1967), and the percentage of the elderly with supplemental policies has grown so that by 1984, 72 percent of the elderly had a supplemental policy (Cafferata, 1985; Rice, 1987). The numbers have not changed much since then, as approximately three-quarters of all Medicare recipients have a supplemental insurance policy (Xu, 2003; Zhang et al., 2009).

The costs of these supplemental policies can vary, and people can change them each year, or choose to add or drop coverage. The best policies may cost many thousands of dollars a year. Not surprisingly, lower-income individuals are less likely to purchase these policies. Of course, if a person's income is low enough or their medical expenses are high enough, they may become eligible for dual coverage (Medicaid in addition to Medicare). In those cases, Medicaid will cover the deductibles and copayments of the Medicare program. Supplemental policies generally cover the deductibles and copayments, but most do not cover services not covered by Medicare. The issue of drug coverage is now a more complex issue with the passage of that expansion to Medicare and is further discussed in Section II of the book. Prior to the passage of the drug coverage, less than half of supplemental plans covered drug costs. Nursing home care is generally not covered by supplemental plans, and people who want such coverage have to purchase separate long-term care insurance policies. Generally, this is also true for coverage of dental care, eyeglasses, and hearing aids. For some of the elderly, supplemental coverage is a benefit of present or past employment and may be similar to insurance purchased prior to retirement. For most others, a number of private health insurance companies provide the insurance coverage, as do elder-advocate groups such as AARP.

Most experts now agree that the development of supplemental plans lessened the political pressure on Congress to expand Medicare benefits. Equity concerns are important as part of supplemental coverage. Besides income, the statuses of race, education, and health are all related to whether a person carries supplemental coverage. For example, whites are twice as likely to have coverage as nonwhites, and the more educated are more likely to have coverage than those with lower levels of education. Slightly less than half of those in poor health have supplemental coverage, while three-quarters of those in excellent health have this coverage. These coverage relationships with social factors help to explain why there is less political pressure to modify and expand Medicare, because the most politically active elderly and those who are most likely to complain to public officials about Medicare problems are more likely to have private supplemental coverage. As previously mentioned in Chapter 2, political activism at all ages is closely linked with socioeconomic status in the United States (Xu, 2003; Zhang et al., 2009).

A third important reason for why there has been little expansion of Medicare benefits is confusion among the elderly about what benefits Medicare does and does not provide. Many elderly are also unsure as to what their supplemental health insurance covers if they have this insurance, and what is left uncovered. Often they do not realize a service is not covered, such as hearing aids, until their hearing begins to decline and they are in need of those services. Because dental and eye care services have generally not been covered (or covered by specialized health insurance plans) during a person's working years, most elderly do not expect those services to be covered by Medicare. Experts do point out that in a more rational system, services that make it possible for people to function in their daily lives (i.e., vision and hearing services) might be considered essential for coverage. (Similarly, in terms of maintaining good health and insuring adequate nutrition, having dental care to retain teeth, or dentures to replace lost teeth, are also important to people as they age.) Probably the most important but uncovered health service, and one that many elderly believe is covered by Medicare, is long-term care. Whether reviewing surveys in the 1980s or the 1990s, generally one-half to one-third of recipients do not realize that Medicare does not cover most long-term care in nursing homes (Oberlander, 2003). In studies of the general public, about one-half think that Medicare will cover the long-term care needs of their older relatives (Oberlander, 2003). Because so many people are confused about what is actually covered by Medicare, it is more difficult for groups such as the AARP to promote interest in these modifications of Medicare benefits.

Beyond these three reasons, the lack of expansion of Medicare benefits is also linked to changes in the administration of the program and to political shifts that occurred in the middle 1990s. Initially, Medicare was administered through the Social Security Administration which was an agency already familiar to many elderly who were used to going to that agency to sign up for Social Security benefits. However, from the earliest days, the actual day-to-day payment of Medicare claims was not part of the responsibility of one government agency, but was given as contracts to various health insurance companies. Blue Cross Blue Shield served this intermediary role in most states. This politically popular arrangement served somewhat to preserve a role for private health insurance companies in running the Medicare program. In addition, the organizational tasks of controlling pension payments that were based upon a set formula was very different from those tasks associated with the oversight of a large number of hospitals and physicians. For ease of implementation, it was faster and less complicated to allow groups, such as private health insurance companies that already had the necessary experience, fulfill those tasks. Thus, the initial legislative mandate of Medicare was to protect the nation's elderly from the economic burdens of illness without significantly interfering with the traditional organization of American medicine.

In 1977, the increasing complexity of Medicare and Medicaid, and the growing costs and size of the programs, led Congress to create a new agency to administer the programs, the Health Care Financing Administration (HCFA). This change moved Medicare out of the Social Security Administration, with its focus on serving the elderly, and into an agency whose focus became the control of health care expenditures with the oversight to assure that providers behaved in appropriate ways. This happened around the same time that the Medicaid Anti-fraud and Abuse amendments were passed that charged the HCFA with collecting and analyzing hospital cost data. Two experts on Medicare, Marmor (2000) and Oberlander (1995) have both argued that this seemingly technical administrative change made possible the implementation of reform of hospital and physician payment in the 1980s. Yet for beneficiaries, the move only compounded difficulties in dealing with Medicare. Social Security offices no longer viewed the administrative issues of Medicare as their concerns, and the elderly received less help in dealing with delays, complicated forms, and questions about payment. Rather than having an actual office to go to for help, most Medicare recipients with reimbursement questions were handled by the toll-free telephone numbers of the fiscal intermediaries that paid Medicare claims.

The continued administrative changes in Medicare have had less actual impact on beneficiaries of Medicare. In 2001, the HCFA, as the agency over Medicare and Medicaid, became known as the Centers for Medicare and Medicaid Services (CMMS). Currently, Medicare, Medicaid, and the State Child Health Insurance Programs (SCHIP) are administered by the Centers for Medicare and Medicaid Service. Through these programs, CMMS now either provides health insurance directly or indirectly to over

74 million Americans. For Medicare, this means that the new agency oversees the performance of the insurance companies that administer Medicare Part A (hospital insurance) and Part B (medical insurance) and pay the providers for services rendered. These organizations are generally called fiscal intermediaries (Part A) and carriers (Part B). CMMS is also responsible for combating fraud and abuse in the Medicare and Medicaid programs, setting national policies for paying health care providers, conducting research on the effectiveness of health care services, and enforcing the policies related to the quality of health care services.

The regulation of clinical laboratories performing tests on patients paid by Medicare also falls under the jurisdiction of CMMS with advice from the Centers for Disease Control (CDC). One current concern is that CMMS is straining to perform its duties, because Congress and the executive branch, regardless of party, have chronically deprived the agency of the necessary managerial resources. There are some fears this might be even more problematic when health care reform is implemented and more responsibilities are added to the agency without a corresponding increase in funding (Executive and Legislative Branches of Both Parties Underfund the Centers for Medicare and Medicaid Services, 2009).

MEDICARE CATASTROPHIC COVERAGE ACT AND ITS REPEAL

One of the most interesting issues related to health care that happened in the late 1980s was the passage and subsequent repeal of the Medicare Catastrophic Coverage Act of 1988 (MCCA). This debate and change in policy helped to reveal the growing connections between interest group politics and Medicare and the new focus upon politics of deficit reduction. In an era of concern over controlling costs and expenditures, the MCCA greatly expanded Medicare's benefits. This expansion of benefits not only occurred while Ronald Reagan was president, but was promoted initially by his administration. This seems anomalous because here was a president interested in both cutting back welfare state programs and concerned about rising health care expenditures.

The personal interest of Otis Bowen, Reagan's Secretary of Health and Human Services, was part of the reason for the passage of the MCCA. Bowen was both a former family physician and former governor of Indiana. From 1982 to 1984, he chaired the federal Advisory Council on Social Security, a group that also reviewed Medicare. This group recommended that Medicare hospitalization coverage be expanded to an unlimited number of days, that the hospital and skilled nursing facility coinsurance requirements be eliminated, and that Medicare beneficiaries be offered an optional Part B benefit (physician services) that would put a cap on out-of-pocket expenses. Bowen sought to enact these changes, and he convinced others in the Reagan administration to go along with them. Some conservatives were pushing a greater emphasis on supplemental health plans as a way to replace more extensive coverage, but Bowen convinced the Reagan administration that his plan was simpler to administer.

Bowen had a greater chance for success because Democrats in Congress were becoming dissatisfied with Medicare's limited coverage of care for chronic conditions (Rovner, 1987). As the new amendment to Medicare was drafted, the benefits under the Medicare Catastrophic Coverage Act (MCCA) were going to be fairly extensive, including not only the recommendations from the Advisory Council mentioned above, but also expanded provisions for hospice care, home health services, mammography screening, outpatient prescription drugs, guaranteed payment of Medicare premiums for impoverished elderly, and protection from impoverishment from nursing home costs of a spouse. One service not covered under the original plan, however, was the coverage of long-term institutionalization in nursing homes. This was a service that many Medicare recipients often erroneously assumed was covered, and therefore, was viewed by many as the most important service to be added to Medicare benefits. Important interest groups such as the AARP and the Villers Foundation (later Families USA) considered a campaign to have long-term care added to Medicare benefits while other groups simply wanted prescription drug coverage. A compromise was reached by adding drug benefits to the bill in place of long-term care insurance.

A separate issue with the proposed MCCA legislation was funding. President Reagan did not want the bill to add to the federal deficit. Increasing the Social Security payroll tax was also viewed as unacceptable, as was a general tax increase. What remained was funding by the elderly themselves, probably through an increase in the Part B premium. Even though the Democrats controlled the House Ways and Means Committee, the principle of self-financing was not challenged. To make it work, a subgroup of beneficiaries, the more affluent elderly, would pay a supplemental premium, with a limit of $800 in 1989. This proposal was supported by an unusual coalition of liberals and conservatives. Conservatives had always disliked the universal aspect of Medicare coverage, and viewed income-related premiums as a way to lessen the government subsidy to wealthy individuals that they felt held back on the purchase of private insurance. Liberals worried more about equity, and that further increases in Part B, which is optional not mandatory, might force low-income people to withdraw from the program. Having a higher payment by higher-income recipients followed the progressive income taxation approach of Social Security in which lower-income retirees receive a higher rate of return on their contributions than do wealthier Social Security contributors.

After the passage of the MCCA, many elderly had a negative reaction both to benefits and costs. Rather than being pleased by the coverage of extended hospitalization, many focused upon the lack of coverage for nursing home care, what many people really considered a catastrophic situation whose financial impact could be disastrous for a family. The affluent elderly became a vocal, organized group with a strong negative reaction to the legislation and the additional costs that had been placed upon them. Groups such as the National Committee to Preserve Social Security and Medicare helped to create an impression that the new legislation required an extra premium from most elderly individuals. Within 16 months, the legislation was repealed by a very large margin (Himmelfarb, 1995; Marmor, 2000; Oberlander, 2003). The repeal of additional benefits still left many unresolved issues for the Medicare program, including no prescription drug coverage, no long-term care coverage, and the lack of coverage of extended hospitalizations. These are some of the important Medicare coverage issues to be addressed in Section II of this book.

Controversies and Issues Related to Medicare

Current Issues in Medicare: Drug Coverage, HMOs/Managed Care Options, and Other Federal Government Programs for Health Care Coverage

This section of the book examines the most important current issues and controversies of the Medicare program. The topics presented in Chapter 4 of this section include prescription drug coverage, HMOs and managed care as part of Medicare, and the link between Medicare and other government programs which provide health care insurance, such as Medicaid and the State Child Health Insurance Program (SCHIP). In Chapter 5 of this section, the initial topics are the lack of long term-care (LTC) and ties with Medicaid as a source of LTC. Chapter 5 continues with a discussion of Medicare and the demographic-based funding crisis and the issues of trust funds as part of Medicare and financing fee schedules. The last part of Chapter 5 presents health care reform, incentives for more universal coverage and the impact of universal coverage upon the operation of Medicare as a program.

Many of the present concerns about Medicare derive from the program's background as enacted in 1965. At that time, Medicare was comparable to the health insurance that many individuals had through their jobs. Although there have been many changes in Medicare, as discussed in Section I of the book and as detailed in the legislative changes in Section III, many aspects of the basic structure have remained such as the separate programs (Part A to cover hospital expenses and Part B to cover physician expenses). Important changes in the past decade include the addition of Part D to cover prescription drug costs and the addition, and impending changes, of managed care or HMOs (health maintenance organizations). Both of these aspects of Medicare are discussed in this chapter as are the other two government programs that provide health insurance coverage and health care to specialized groups: Medicaid, which passed at the same time as Medicare, and State Child Health Insurance Programs (SCHIP), passed in 1996. Medicaid, although initially conceived as a program for poor mothers and their children, is now also a program that covers certain costs for the elderly who meet income qualifications.

THE PRESCRIPTION DRUG COVERAGE ADDITION TO MEDICARE

The addition of prescription drug coverage to the Medicare program was passed at the end of President George W. Bush's first term as president. The program was a political compromise between Congressional Democrats and Republicans, all of whom wanted to return to their home states and districts and claim success in improving Medicare as they ran for reelection. In 2003, the Medicare Prescription Drug, Improvement, and Modernization Act of 2003 (MMA) was passed by the House (220–215) and the Senate (54–44) in November and signed into law (Public Law 108-173) by President Bush in December. This Law provided a new outpatient prescription drug benefit under Medicare beginning in 2006. In the interim, it also created a temporary prescription drug discount card and transitional assistance program called the Medicare-Approved Drug Discount Card Program, begun in 2004 as a transition to the new drug program. In 2004 and 2005, another transitional program provided a $600 annual credit to low-income Medicare beneficiaries who were without prescription drug coverage. These transitional programs were beneficial to some beneficiaries, but they were very confusing to the elderly. It took people time to first understand the new temporary program, and then, to understand and enroll in the new drug program. In addition to the major drug benefit aspect of this bill, the MMA also made other important changes in Medicare. These included establishing a new income-related Part B premium for beneficiaries with higher incomes (beginning in 2007), indexing the Part B deductible and creating some changes to the Medicare HMO plans, known before this legislation as Medicare + Choice and now called the Medicare Advantage program.

The passage of the Part D Drug Option was a major addition to the Medicare program and partially addressed what had been a major criticism—the lack of drug coverage. Studies prior to the passage of this program have documented the impact upon beneficiaries of the lack of drug coverage in the Medicare program. Xu (2003), in an important article in the journal *Health Affairs*, examined cross-sectional differences in the financial burden of prescription drug use among U.S. elderly and nonelderly adult populations. Xu used data from the 1998 Medical Expenditure Panel Survey to compare out-of-pocket spending for prescriptions, copayment rates, and the proportion of family income spent on prescription drugs by elderly people with working-age adults. Even after adjusting for utilization or need, financial differences were still observed between elderly and nonelderly adult populations. Comparisons showed that the elderly at 200–399 percent of the poverty level paid $298 more out-of-pocket for prescription drugs than their non-elderly cohorts. Those in the poorest group (below 100 percent of the federal poverty level) paid only $133 more. Differences between elderly and nonelderly consumers' income proportion was the greatest for the near-poor (100–124% of poverty) and low-income (125–199% of poverty) groups. In particular, lower-income elderly people were worse off than were nonelderly adults in the same poverty class and their elderly peers in other poverty classes.

Other studies employed different data, such as the Medicare Current Beneficiary Survey. The data is culled from 11,000 interviews with Medicare recipients to learn more about their experience of Medicare and issues that develop with the use of Medicare services. Generally, Medicare beneficiaries who do not have prescription drug coverage are less likely to fill prescriptions and end up with higher out-of-pocket drug expenditures than beneficiaries with coverage (through a privately purchased supplemental plan or through an employer based plan that continued to provide some coverage to retirees as a supplement to Medicare). Prior to the enactment of the Part D drug benefit, approximately one-third of the elderly had no drug coverage, had higher out-of-pocket costs, and were also less likely to fill prescriptions. Even a cost for a specific drug might be higher than that paid by younger people with drug coverage through an employer-based plan or by retirees with certain drug coverage, because some health insurance plans negotiate reduced fees for drugs. However, Medicare beneficiaries without any drug coverage generally did not receive the discounts given to large insurers.

As previously mentioned, Medicare Part D is a prescription drug insurance plan that provides beneficiaries with prescription drug benefits. To receive these benefits, a monthly premium must be paid annually, and failure to pay will result in an interruption of coverage. People must choose among available plans in their state. The costs for the plans vary, as do the specifics of drugs that are covered, which potentially make the choices confusing to consumers—an initial concern with the program. Because not every plan will cover the same drugs, people must search current medications for coverage under the available Medicare Part D plans in their state. Although consumers were initially confused, most are now choosing to enroll in a plan, unless they have supplemental coverage through a retirement work-based plan or other supplemental plan that provides similar drug coverage as the typical Part D plan. The Medicare.gov Web site provides many tools to help people determine which plans are best for them, including ways to compare

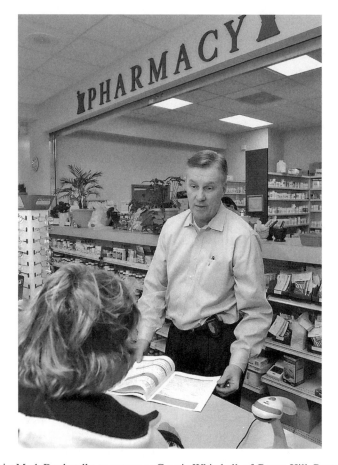

Pharmacist Mark Doyle talks to customer Connie Whitehall, of Centre Hill, Pennsylvania, about her mother's prescription drug plan options, January 18, 2006. Following passage of Medicare Part D on January 1st, pharmacists had to help customers deal with the complexities of the new drug benefit program. (AP Photo/Pat Little)

the drug formularies of different plans against their current medications. Even with these improvements, there is little question that the need to separately choose a drug plan, while a helpful benefit to most of the elderly, brings with it complications.

Selecting a plan is also difficult for some of the elderly who require help from family or friends who are more familiar with using computers to research health care options. As part of the Part D legislation, employers or plans that administer retiree drug coverage are required to provide information (a creditable coverage disclosure notice) about whether the retiree health or drug coverage will be affected upon joining a Medicare drug plan. This information must tell a person how the retiree drug coverage compares to the new Medicare prescription drug coverage. If the retiree drug coverage will remain the same, and the coverage is creditable (it expects to pay, on average, at least as much as Medicare coverage), a person can stay with existing coverage, and not have to pay a penalty for a later change to Medicare drug coverage. All of these aspects increase the complexity of Part D, making it a more complicated experience for Medicare beneficiaries than the experience with Part A and Part B.

Medicare Part D uses a tier-based system to determine pricing and eligibility for prescription drugs. Each tier is priced at a pre-determined price bracket and/or copayment assignment. These fluctuate depending upon income level, as well as plan type. All plans cover both brand name and generic prescription drugs and are accepted at most U.S. pharmacies. Medicare Part D plans must cover all, or substantially all, drugs in six categories: antidepressants, antipsychotics, anti-convulsants, anti-retrovirals (AIDS treatment), immune-suppressants, and anti-cancer. As an example, the 2006 criteria established by the Centers for Medicare and Medicaid Services (CMS), the federal agency that administers both Medicare and Medicaid, was that there had to be 75 percent coverage for medications after an annual deductible of $250 until $2,500 in drug costs was reached, and 95 percent coverage for the rest of the calendar year after $5,100 in total expenditures. Most people on Medicare choose a plan through a stand-alone prescription drug plan (PDP), which is how Part D works for most, although people in the managed care option of Medicare Advantage plans also use those managed care plans for drug coverage.

The coverage gap in Medicare Part D which is the lack of coverage between $2,500 and $5,100 has become known as the coverage gap or "donut hole." When a beneficiary spends between $2,500 and $5,100 on covered medications, plans are not required to provide any coverage. There are some plans that do provide minimal coverage in this range, but they mostly cover only generic drugs. In general, patients may have to pay 100 percent out-of-pocket for all their drugs in this expenditure range or for all non-generic drugs. The "donut hole" was created as a way to provide a large amount of coverage (75%) to most Medicare beneficiaries after the modest deductible, but also not be too expensive to maintain throughout the year. For those with extremely high drug costs, catastrophic coverage resumes and covers the rest of their drug expenditures in that year. This "donut hole" has become one of the most controversial aspects of the Part D plan. Another controversial aspect is that the federal government is not allowed to negotiate drug prices for Medicare, as it does on behalf of the Veteran's Administration and Medicaid.

After what most Medicare experts would describe as a difficult beginning caused by the confusion encountered in learning about this new program and its many options, how well is Part D prescription coverage working? This is an especially important question because this part of Medicare coverage is organized as a market in which consumers will choose among different plans offered competitively by many insurance companies and HMOs. In an assessment by the Nobel-winning economist Daniel McFadden (2007), he argues that after the initial confusion, people did participate in the program, with only 7.4 percent of the 65 and over eligible population not enrolling in Part D or in a comparable prescription drug coverage plan. Average premiums, initially estimated to be around $37 a month, were actually lower. Because enrollment is voluntary, there were still about 1.2 million elderly, primarily poorly educated elderly above the poverty line, who use enough prescription drugs to benefit from this coverage, but chose not to enroll. McFadden (2007) argues, however, that consumers were fairly consistent in understanding their own needs, and in selecting the lowest cost plan that provided good coverage given their health problems. He also stresses that one reason for this consumer success was active management within Medicare, which worked hard to ensure that all plans were adequate and that consumers had ways to find out detailed information about the availability of drugs under different plans. These efforts made the innately confusing process easier to understand and helped beneficiaries to figure out which plans would work best for them.

Several recent articles published in the journal *Health Affairs* examined the effect of Medicare Part D coverage on drug use and cost sharing (Schneeweiss, Patrick, Pedan, Varasteh, Levin, Liu, and Shrank, 2009) and the effects of the coverage gap on drug spending in Medicare Part D (Zhang, Donohue, Newhouse, and Lave, 2009). Schneeweiss and his colleagues found that use of some drugs, such as statins which treat high cholesterol, stabilized at levels 11 to 37 percent above the trend in usage that would have been expected without participation in Part D of Medicare. A negative finding is that when beneficiaries reached the "donut hole," about 12 percent would decrease essential medication usage. Zhang and his colleagues report a similar finding in their study, citing that those lacking coverage for drugs in the "donut hole" period reduced their drug use by 14 percent. The proportion of beneficiaries reaching the "donut hole" increased as the number of chronic conditions of a beneficiary increased.

Another evaluation of the Part D drug benefit was conducted by Fisher and Rosenberg (2007) and included a detailed literature review of previously published articles about Part D. It also included an independent analysis of medication costs that would be covered by Part D through modeling prescription expenditures of the eligible population, using consumer data available from the Medicare Current Beneficiary Survey. After reviewing some operational aspects of the program, which they argue began to improve as public understanding of some of the details increased, Fisher and Rosenberg estimated an expenditure of $1,331 per beneficiary in insurance-covered drug expenditures, and a ten-year expenditure estimate of $520 billion. The latter is comparable to the projection of the Centers for Medicare and Medicaid Services of $534 billion, but is larger than the amount accepted by Congress when the bill was passed, leading to concerns about the future of the drug benefit and Medicare, and the belief by Fisher and Rosenberg that cost reforms will eventually be necessary.

The newly passed 2010 health care reform legislation does address the issue of the "donut hole" in the Medicare drug plans. The phase-out of the "donut hole" will begin with a $250 rebate to Medicare beneficiaries who hit the coverage gap in 2010. Beginning in 2011, there will be a 50 percent discount on brand-name drugs in the "donut hole" for people with incomes below $85,000 per individual and $170,000 per couple. Eventually, the "donut hole" will be closed by 2020 by increasing the discount until the benefit reaches 75 percent of the cost. For higher-income recipients, the cost of both Part B and Part D to them will be increased, although the exact details are not yet clear.

MEDICARE AND HMO/MANAGED CARE OPTIONS

In 1997, the Balanced Budget Act gave Medicare recipients the option of receiving their benefits through private managed care, then called Medicare + Choice Plans, or through regular Medicare, which is the traditional fee-for-service program. This Act authorized local preferred provider organizations (PPOs) as well as medical savings accounts and the establishment of a payment floor, mostly applicable to rural counties. This was not the first Medicare option related to health maintenance organizations (HMOs) or managed care as they later became known. The Balanced Budget Act replaced the Medicare Risk contract program, also known as section 1876 of the Social Security Act. That program was authorized in 1982 as part of the Tax Equity and Fiscal Responsibility Act, which built upon a provision that had been started in the 1970s. This allowed private plans to contract with Medicare for reimbursement of costs for providing care to Medicare beneficiaries. Not all the plans that had operated under the risk contract provisions decided to participate in Medicare + Choice, which started in 1999. Of the 346 contracts in place in 1999, 45 withdrew and another 54 reduced the areas they were willing to serve (Morgan, Smith, and Chaikind, 2003).

Further changes, improvements, and modifications were passed as part of the Benefits Improvement and Protection Act of 2000 (BIPA). This enhanced payments by creating payment floors for urban areas, and also increasing the floor for rural areas and the Medicare Modernization Act of 2003 (MMA). The MMA renamed the program "Medicare Advantage," authorized two additional plan types (regional PPOs and special needs plans), and boosted payments to encourage plan participation. The Medicare Improvements for Patients and Providers Act (MIPPA) of 2008 included changes in payments to plans, and added beneficiary protections, focusing on marketing practices.

Today, the private managed care option is called Medicare Advantage and provides health plan options that are approved by Medicare and run by private companies, but are still under the overall approval of the Medicare program. If a beneficiary chooses to participate in a Medicare Advantage plan, the person will receive all of their Medicare-covered health care through this plan. Generally, this will include doctor visits, hospital visits, and often, prescription drug coverage. Some plans offer extra benefits such as coverage for vision, hearing, and dental problems; this class of care is not covered by regular Medicare. Often the out-of-pocket costs for such plans may be less than regular Medicare without buying a Medigap policy.

Interest in the HMO/PPO options under Medicare has been increasing in recent years, after a slow start to the program. In 2009, the majority of the 45 million people on Medicare are in the fee-for-service (FFS) version of Medicare; however, 22 percent are also now enrolled in a private Medicare Advantage plan. This is an increase from earlier years. Since 2003, the number of Medicare beneficiaries enrolled in private plans has nearly doubled from 5.3 million in 2003 to the current level of 10.2 million (Kaiser Family Foundation, 2009).

The 1997 legislation that resulted in the Medicare + Choice plans was the result of the failure of some earlier attempts to modify either Medicare or health care in general. After the failure of the Clinton health care reform plan in 1993–1994, and continued rising costs in Medicare in the 1990s

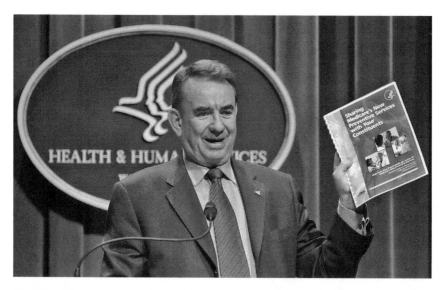

Health and Human Services secretary Tommy Thompson, shows a *Medicare's Preventive Services* pamphlet during a press conference, January 10, 2005, in Washington, D.C. Thompson talked about the Medicare Modernization Act benefits and new education and outreach efforts. (AP Photo/Manuel Balce Ceneta)

following the payment reform efforts of PPS for hospital payment and RBRVS for physician payment, Republicans who controlled Congress in 1995 became interested in modifying Medicare's budgetary entitlement status. As an entitlement program, the costs of Medicare must be met each year, and there is no overall cap, for example, on the total amount of dollars that can be spent on Medicare in a given year. Republicans in Congress were interested in a cap on health expenditures that eventually would convert the Medicare fee-for-service program into a defined contribution or voucher type plan. In a defined contribution plan, people who purchase the insurance are covered for expenses up to a set dollar limit for each expense. In a voucher plan, people would receive a voucher for a set dollar amount to be used to purchase insurance through the private marketplace. In some small businesses, for example, employers will provide a voucher amount that the employee can then use to purchase health insurance from other companies that are in business in the area, rather than dealing with the creation of a health insurance plan for employees.

Republicans in Congress wanted to provide services to current Medicare beneficiaries through private insurance plans. They hoped that this would increase the enrollment of people over the age of 65 in managed care. Republicans embraced this plan because denying services currently available with the fee-for-service program was politically unpopular, but the idea of weaning the elderly from the original program into managed care options remained a goal, along with strict limits on overall spending. President Clinton and the Democrats in Congress opposed these reforms and although legislation was passed in 1995 on an almost exclusively partisan vote, President Clinton vetoed the legislation. These party differences on Medicare became part of the 1996 presidential campaign in which President Clinton defeated the Republican candidate Bob Dole.

By 1997, however, concerns about rising costs and an interest in HMOs as a way to reform part of Medicare were still issues. This resulted in the passage of the Balanced Budget Act of 1997 that made a number of changes in Medicare, including encouraging HMO options. The Act was met with bipartisan support. For Republicans and the managed care industry, the 1997 reforms were a step toward the possibility of transforming Medicare into a competitive market in which more people on Medicare would purchase insurance through private plans as their Medicare options. For Democrats, the reforms retained a commitment to the Medicare fee-for-service option in that beneficiaries would not be financially penalized for staying in the traditional Medicare option.

Both political parties realized that deficit pressures in the program were real and that Medicare-spending reductions would be important in order to have a balanced federal budget. Some health policy experts did view this change as the beginning of a transition from a single payer system to the creation of a health insurance market for Medicare (Christensen, 1998).

At the time, managed care was becoming a dominant model in the U.S. health care industry, and the new legislation extended that optimism about the benefits of managed care to those participants in the Medicare program who elected to participate in the HMO option. During the planning for this program, the estimates from the Congressional Budget Office were that 27 percent of Medicare beneficiaries would pick the Medicare + Choice plans in 2002 and 35 percent by 2005 (Christensen, 1998). However, these estimates were much higher than actually occurred. Only 11 percent of beneficiaries were in an HMO type plan in 2004 and in 2009, while the percentage has been increasing, the figure was still lower (22% of current Medicare enrollees in 2009 picked a Medicare Advantage plan) than the CBO estimate for 2002 (Kaiser Family Foundation, 2009).

There are currently some advantages to being enrolled in the Medicare Advantage plans. According to Medicare, if you register with one of these plans, you do not need to purchase a Medigap policy, and you may have lower out-of-pocket costs. In exchange for this option, a person will generally have restricted choice in physicians and hospitals. There are five unique plans that fall under this category including HMO, Preferred Provider Organizations, Private Fee-for-Service plans, Medicare Special Needs plans, and Medicare Medical Savings Account plans. HMO plans have been available through Medicare since the 1970s while the other plans were created in the legislation passed in 1997 and 2003. The number of Medicare beneficiaries enrolled in these private plans has been steadily increasing from 5.3 million in 2003 to 8.7 million in 2007 and to 10.2 million in 2009 (Kaiser Family Foundation, 2009). The majority of people in this option are enrolled in the HMO plans.

The introduction of the Medicare + Choice option to the public was not particularly easy. Because the payments to plans varied across geographic areas, this was both confusing to Medicare recipients and meant that plans in high-payment areas often offered generous benefits above those provided in traditional Private Fee-for-Service (PFFS) Medicare. In low-cost areas, there were often no additional benefits beyond those provided by PFFS Medicare. Also, in the late 1990s, plans sometimes began participating in Medicare and then decided not to continue, resulting both in enrollees having to enroll in another plan or switch to traditional PFFS Medicare and decreased public interest in the program. Many who lived in rural areas never had the choice of an HMO plan in which to participate. Some options that might have been more attractive to Medicare recipients, such as the private fee-for-service (PFFS) plans which would have allowed the freedom to choose any provider, were never fully developed and were also not realistic options for many. By 2003, only Sterling Life Insurance Company was offering a Medicare PFFS plan, and it was available in only about half of the counties in the United States which represented 38 percent of all Medicare beneficiaries (Colamery, 2003; Morgan and Smith, 2003).

The issue of providers leaving the Medicare + Choice program presented a serious drawback. In September 2001, Medicare announced that 536,000 beneficiaries enrolled in Medicare + Choice would have to change their coverage by January 2002. In 2002, 22 plans that had been operational with Medicare in 2001 left the program, and another 36 reduced the geographic areas they were willing to serve. Between 1999 and 2002, between 5 to 15 percent of participating plans withdrew each year (Morgan, Smith, and Chaikind, 2003). Plan administrators argued that they withdrew due to inadequate payments, increased regulatory burden, and the difficulty in the development and maintenance of a provider network. Some health care experts argue that financial instability is one reason that some Medicare plans withdrew, as they have often been smaller plans and plans newer to the provision of managed care. Other experts point out that withdrawing from delivery of services and the consolidation of plans has also occurred in the overall managed care market, not just in the Medicare market (Colamery, 2003; Morgan and Smith, 2003). This may be a correction to the rapid growth in managed care within the health care market in the mid-1990s.

A number of studies have compared Medicare fee-for-service and managed care plans focusing on differences in quality of care. Medicare managed care plans overall did not appear to offer an equally high quality of care when compared to Medicare fee-for-service plans (regular Medicare). Referral rates, the rate of inpatient versus outpatient care, and the length of hospital visits were all lower in managed care plans (Wong and Hellinger, 2001). One study reported that managed care enrollees were less likely to receive needed coronary angiography, a potentially lifesaving procedure, after the experience of a heart attack (AHRQ, 2000). Another study compared outcomes among chronically ill Medicare beneficiaries in fee-for-service and managed care plans (Ware, Bayliss, Rogers, Kosinski, and Tarlov, 1996), and found managed care enrollees experienced greater declines in physical health as compared to fee-for-service enrollees. The same study also reported that those living in poverty had better physical and mental health outcomes in fee-for-service plans, although those living above the poverty line experienced better outcomes in managed care plans (Ware et al., 1996).

Another aspect of quality of care is the use of preventive care and managed care Medicare plans look better by this measure. Several studies have documented increased attention to preventive care among some Medicare managed care plans (Miller and Luft, 1994; Schneider, Cleary, Zaslavsky, and Epstein, 2001; Greene, Blustein, and Laflamme, 2001; Landon, Zaslavsky, Bernard, Cioffi, and Cleary, 2004). There is, however, much regional variation in the provision of preventive care by managed care plans (Moran, 1999).

Hacker (2003) argued Medicare reform needs to be universal (i.e., for all Medicare enrollees), as opposed to only lodged within managed care.

This option would be more costly for the federal government, but it would equate to a policy that benefits all older adults equally, rich and poor as well as the sick and healthy, while keeping in line Medicare's original approach as a social insurance program. By 2003, a number of experts on Medicare such as Jonathan Oberlander (2003) were concluding that Medicare + Choice was a policy failure due to declining enrollment and an array of other problems already mentioned. Some of this lack of enthusiasm was related to the overall private health insurance market, in which premium increases for health insurance had returned to the double-digit inflation rates of the 1980s. Instead of controlling health care costs, managed care now simply appeared to be another sector experiencing rapidly increased costs, making Medicare managed care no longer an attractive option financially for many beneficiaries. This held true even for Congressional conservatives who, in theory, preferred the introduction of more private market mechanisms into Medicare. Although the numbers of enrollees have been increasing, enrollment rates in managed care Medicare plans vary greatly across the United States. Enrollment rates are substantially higher in urban (25%) than in rural (13%) counties, but there is a great deal of state-by-state variation. Some states have less than 10 percent of the Medicare population in the Advantage plan whereas 12 states and the District of Columbia enroll more than 30 percent of Medicare recipients in an Advantage plan (Kaiser Family Foundation, 2009). Currently, Medicare Advantage plans are paid more per recipient than the average costs for Medicare recipients in the PFFS program in the same area. These higher costs raise issues of equity and have led some policy analysts to believe that the Advantage options are generally not a good idea for the Medicare program.

Two recent discussions of the Medicare Advantage program tend to support the concern about whether private health insurance plans as part of Medicare Advantage are really better for beneficiaries or for the overall heath and stability of the Medicare program. Berenson and Down (2009) conclude that assuring stable plan choices and providing extra benefits in these plans ends up costing extra money for Medicare, meaning that Medicare is actually paying more dollars each year for care for those enrolled in Medicare Advantage plans. These additional costs weaken the financial stability of Medicare overall, while contributing to inequities across beneficiary groups. Berenson and Down believe that policymakers should focus on leveling the public-private "playing field," and deal with fiscal issues, rather than push for more expansion of Medicare Advantage plans. Gold (2009) conducted a review of plans, using both quantitative program data and qualitative data from telephone interviews with 19 plan sponsors that enroll over 3.5 million participants. From both data sources, she concludes that the changes of the Medicare Modernization Act has expanded choice and the private sector role, but has also added to Medicare's complexity and costs and has created potential inequities. At a minimum, Gold believes that a stronger system of performance monitoring and greater oversight responsibilities over the Medicare program are required.

Changes will occur in the Medicare Advantage program as a part of recent health care reform. The Obama administration has targeted changes in the Medicare Advantage program prior to the more detailed discussion of health care reform. There was already a proposal to try and save $177 billion over ten years through a new competitive-bidding system for Medicare Advantage plans. In 2009, these private plans received an average 14 percent—or $12 billion—more than the government would pay if beneficiaries enrolled in those plans had remained in the traditional Medicare program. The Obama administration's initial plan would have gone beyond other proposals to cut payments to Medicare Advantage plans. Under the initial proposal, companies in a given geographic area would submit bids to cover Medicare beneficiaries, as they do now, but they would be paid the average of their bids, plus some additional amounts. Insurers submitting below-average bids would receive the average payment; they could then use the difference between their bids and the average payment amount to provide additional benefits to enrollees. Companies with above-average bids would charge members a premium to make up the shortfall between the average payment and their bids (Jaffe, 2009).

The 2010 health reform legislation also reduces Medicare payments to the Medicare Advantage plans. The legislation will make payments to Advantage plans equal (on average, per beneficiary) to payments through traditional Medicare. Up to this point in time, Medicare Advantage plans have received $135 on average more per beneficiary per month than the traditional fee-for-service Medicare. Although the legislation will cut payments, there are no provisions for cuts to mandated benefits. To deal with the reduction in payments, plans may cut extra, optional benefits such as vision and dental care. The provisions for equalizing payments between Medicare Advantage plans and traditional Medicare are based on a recommendation by the non-partisan Medicare Payment Advisory Commission (MedPAC), and supported by advocates for Medicare beneficiaries such as the Center for Medicare Advocacy. One purpose of these provisions is to extend the life of the Medicare Trust Fund which, without some intervention, is projected to be depleted in 2017. These provisions will result in approximately $118 billion in savings. There are some "sweeteners" for plans that perform well; there could be a 2 percent bonus for plans which offer specified care coordination benefits and up to an additional 4 percent bonus if their quality is highly rated according to the Centers for Medicare and Medicaid Services (CMS) star-rating system.

OTHER GOVERNMENT PROGRAMS FOR HEALTH CARE LESS FOCUSED ON THE ELDERLY

Medicaid and State Child Health Insurance Programs (SCHIP) are two other large government programs that provide health care services to selected groups in the population. Although this book is primarily about Medicare, the health care program for the elderly and those who qualify for disability payments under Social Security, it is important for readers to understand these two other major federal programs that provide health care services. Medicaid legislation was passed at the same time that Medicare legislation was passed, in 1965. At that time, it was created as a program to provide health benefits to poor individuals who qualified for welfare payments. In contrast to Medicare, which is a federal program with similar benefits across states, Medicaid is a joint state-federal entitlement program administered by states under broad federal guidelines. The costs for the program are shared between states and the federal government. Not all of the poor are covered by the program, and how this works has varied over time. When the Medicaid was first created, children and their mothers who were recipients of AFDC (Aid to Families of Dependent Children) were the major recipients of care through this program, and receipt of care was tied to eligibility for the various categorical welfare programs which, as with Medicaid, are joint state-federal programs. One complication is that states can vary the eligibility levels for welfare eligibility, which meant that access to Medicaid also varied greatly from state to state. While the federal government pays an average of 55 percent of the costs, its share can range from 50 to 80 percent, depending upon a state's per capita income.

Over the past 25 years, Congress has mandated coverage up to higher income levels for some groups and specified coverage for certain other groups. There have also been cuts in Medicaid matching funds starting with the Reagan administration in the early 1980s. In 1981, 1982, and 1983, federal matching funds were reduced by 3, 4, and 4.5 percent respectively for the upcoming fiscal years. As a way to allow some experimentation, states no longer had to provide free choice of providers in Medicaid and could begin managed care programs. States were also allowed to require small copays for some basic services provided to some of the Medicaid population. All of these changes lowered or modified benefits to Medicaid recipients. In contrast, other changes expanded the number of groups who were eligible to receive benefits which began with mandates for coverage of pregnant women and young children in the early 1980s. The Omnibus Budget and Reconciliation Act of 1989 mandated that, beginning in April 1990, states had to cover pregnant women and children under the age of six with family incomes up to 133 percent of the federal poverty level. In 1988, Congress mandated that states continue Medicaid coverage for one year for beneficiaries who lose their eligibility for the program as their income increases. These and later mandates have meant that costs for Medicaid for states have increased, so that in many states, one of the largest single budget items is the Medicaid match.

Another major expansion was the Omnibus Budget and Reconciliation Act of 1990 that mandated coverage for all children 6 through 18 years of age in families whose incomes were below the federal poverty level. This portion of the population would receive that benefit whether or not they also received AFDC cash assistance. This was covered with a plan that was phased in a year at a time and completed by 2002. Despite these increases in costs and coverage in the program, not all those individuals with low incomes are covered. Children have been one group with better coverage rates, and this is even truer now with the SCHIP program, discussed in more detail in the following paragraphs. Medicaid, however, often does not cover the working poor or those who may work at a job and barely earn an income above the poverty level. The federal portion of the program does not cover most adults in this situation, although states can decide to cover this group which is often related to overall state tax revenues. In 2008 and 2009, when

Erica Collins talks about her daughter, Kayla, January 11, 2007, at Rainbow Babies & Children's Hospital, in Cleveland. Collins, who had spent much of the previous night with her premature baby at Rainbow Hospital, made a brief appearance at the local forum to encourage parents to sign up their children for State Children's Health Insurance Program (SCHIP), coverage which has helped her family. (AP Photo/Tony Dejak)

many states were having a very difficult time balancing their budgets, some eliminated adults from Medicaid coverage, even though the need was great.

Over the past 15 years, when Republicans were in control of Congress, there was a drive to convert Medicaid into a block grant to states. President Clinton vetoed this legislation in 1995 after it was passed by Congress. This was during a period of concern about the growth of welfare entitlement programs, both AFDC and Medicaid. In 1996, the Personal Responsibility and Work Opportunity Act of 1996 (PRWOA) repealed the AFDC individual entitlement to cash assistance and replaced it with the Temporary Assistance for Needy Families (TANF) block grant to states, thus ending the formal link between cash assistance (welfare) and Medicaid eligibility. PRWOA also required states to cover families that met July 16, 1996 AFDC eligibility standards and allowed states to cover families with higher incomes. The Act also placed a limitation on the availability of Medicaid coverage for non-emergency services to otherwise eligible legal immigrants that had entered the United States on, or after August 22, 1996. The ban was for five years, and after that states could decide on whether to allow coverage for these immigrants.

The Balanced Budget Act of 1997 established the State Children's Health Insurance Program (SCHIP) which allowed states to cover uninsured children in families with incomes below 200 percent of the federal poverty level (FPL) and who were ineligible for Medicaid. The federal funds are capped, but the matching rate for costs of SCHIP services is enhanced (30% higher than state's Medicaid matching rate), with a federal match of 65 percent as a floor and 85 percent as a ceiling. This program was particularly aimed at children of the working poor, a group which often includes parents who are in the labor force but work for an employer who does not provide health care insurance. The number of these parents was expected to increase in future years, as welfare reforms both decreased the number of parents of children formerly on welfare who were receiving cash benefits and increased the number of these people who accept jobs that lack the full set of benefits common to many white-collar and middle-income jobs.

In the five years from fiscal year 1998 onward, $24 billion became available to cover health care for U.S. children. Some sources estimated that free or low cost health care could be provided to up to half of the nation's uninsured children (Rosenbaum et al., 1998). SCHIP is a federal grant-in-aid program that entitles states to elect to participate in federal allotments to targeted low-income children who are ineligible for other insurance coverage, including Medicaid (Rosenbaum, Johnson, Sonosky, Markus, and DeGraw, 1998). The SCHIP program allows states to vary their programs, and some states did not begin the program right away. The SCHIP program started in fiscal year 1998 in some states and in the next fiscal year in others. Moreover, since the SCHIP program follows in the tradition that dictates means-tested welfare programs are joint efforts between state and federal government, there is not just one national SCHIP program, but 50 different SCHIP programs, one for each state. This structural criticism has also been leveled at Medicaid as there is not just one national Medicaid program in the United States.

As previous studies have pointed out, certain groups of children are less likely to be covered by the Medicaid program or have health insurance (Cassil, 1997; Selden et al., 1998; and Davidoff et al., 2000). A common misperception of the U.S. public has been that all poor children receive Medicaid. One reason that many poor children are not enrolled with Medicaid is that parents do not always complete the paperwork to qualify their children. There are a variety of proof of income that are required which may necessitate many time-consuming visits to welfare agencies. This lengthy and complicated qualification process is just one reason why many poor children may not be actually enrolled in the program. One study has estimated that about 30 percent of uninsured children were eligible for Medicaid but not enrolled in 1995. The rest of the children, while uninsured, were not Medicaid eligible (Cassil, 1997). Other studies of children who are eligible for Medicaid, but have not been enrolled, have concluded that at least one of every five children eligible for Medicaid coverage before implementation of the SCHIP program was medically uninsured and that these Medicaid-eligible children accounted for up to one-quarter of all uninsured children. This was despite state outreach and enrollment initiatives (Selden, Banthin, and Cohen, 1998; Davidoff, Garrett, Makuc, and Schirmer, 2000). Children who live outside of metropolitan areas are more likely to be uninsured, as are children who live in the southern and western parts of the United States (Weinick, Weigers, and Cohen, 1998).

One limitation for enrollment for some parents is the cost-sharing feature of the legislation. States can opt to include cost-sharing features either in the forms of premiums for health insurance for families, or as copayments at the time services are received. Twenty-five states have such features, with 12 using both premiums and copayments, 7 using only premiums, and the remaining 6 states engaging in more complicated processes (O'Brien, Archdeacon Barrett, Crow, Janicki, Rousseau, and Williams, 2000). Premium payments provide both enrollment and logistical difficulties, especially because many poor families live in a "cash economy" and have difficulty sending in monthly premium payments. Keeping up with these premiums was also difficult for administration of the program in many states. Copayments created fewer complications for program administrators, but were more annoying to providers of care who had to collect the fees.

Despite all these limitations, SCHIP is having some success in improving the health insurance levels and hence, quality of health, of children. By 1999, 86 percent of children had health coverage, a small increase from 85 percent in 1998, and leading to the lowest rates of no insurance coverage for children since 1993. By 1999, 23 percent of children were covered by public programs such as Medicaid and SCHIP, as compared with only 11 percent in 1987, before SCHIP and some of the Medicaid expansions were instituted (Federal Interagency Forum on Child and Family Statistics, 2001). However, issues of ethnic and racial equity do remain, as 91 percent of white children had either private or government insurance in 1999, versus only 82 percent of African American children and 73 percent of Hispanic children (Kronenfeld, 2002; Kronenfeld, 2006).

Currently, Medicaid and SCHIP play a crucial role in providing health insurance for low-income children from families below 200 percent of the federal poverty level. About half of the 33.2 million low-income children receive coverage from public programs, while 29 percent of low-income children have private coverage. Most children with public coverage are in the Medicaid program (28 million) and six million are covered through SCHIP which leaves nine million children uninsured in the United States. These figures make both Medicaid and SCHIP essential health care safety nets for millions of low-income children. Children represent nearly half of all Medicaid enrollees, but account for only 17 percent of total program spending. The cost to the taxpayer of covering children through Medicaid is relatively inexpensive ($1,410 per child), compared to the much higher Medicaid costs for those adults who use long-term care services. The costs are much lower even though Medicaid pays for a comprehensive set of services for children, including physician and hospital visits, screening and treatment (EPSDT), well-child care, vision care, and dental services (Kaiser Family Fund, 2007). Although at the end of the George W. Bush administration, there were delays in reauthorizing SCHIP legislation, and the program was continued through a resolution mechanism, one of the earliest pieces of legislation passed in the Obama administration was a reauthorization of SCHIP legislation.

One problem with Medicaid today is that there has been growth in spending in recent years. Costs went from about $205 billion in 2000 to about $330 billion in 2007 (Holohan and Yemane, 2009). These costs are a concern because the growth in Medicaid spending has been at a much higher rate than the increase in overall national health spending. Much of the rising costs can be explained by increased enrollment in Medicaid. If costs are considered per enrollee, Medicaid spending actually compares favorably both to increases in medical care prices and gross domestic product. Some of the explanations as to how Medicaid costs have been increasing link to Medicare, and will be one of the topics of consideration in the next chapter. Between 2000 and 2007, Medicaid enrollment increased from 31.8 million people to 42.3 million people, an annual rate of increase of 4.2 percent. Some of this increase is for the aged and disabled, who are typically also enrolled in Medicare, and some of this increase is for children and nondisabled adults. The annual rate of increase among children and nondisabled adults in this time period was 4.9 percent, but the annual rate of increase for the elderly and disabled was a smaller 2.6 percent. Although the rate of increase among the elderly and disabled was slower, the cost impact is not necessarily smaller because the elderly and disabled population have more costly health needs than the younger population on Medicaid. This raises the issue of long-term care coverage, one of the more complex issues impacting both Medicaid and Medicare, and also one of the topics of the next chapter.

CHAPTER 5

Long-term Care Coverage, Medicare and the Demographic-based Funding Crisis, and Health Care Reform

This chapter will focus on several major areas of concern either for the Medicare program itself and how well the program will work in the future or for aspects of the program that leave uncovered areas of need for Medicare recipients. These are critical issues about future concerns for Medicare and what may guide the future changes of the program. The first issue, long-term care coverage, represents care that is presently not well covered by Medicare, but is of paramount importance to many Medicare recipients. The second issue examines both the ensuing demographic-based funding crisis for Medicare, and trust funds and how they tie in to the overall financing of Medicare. The last section of this chapter will focus upon the future of Medicare, and how it specifically relates to the upcoming changes within President Obama's health care reform legislation.

LACK OF LONG-TERM CARE COVERAGE IN MEDICARE

One of the most important services lacking in Medicare is the coverage of long-term care needs for the elderly. It is one of the aspects of the Medicare program that is most misunderstood by the general public and even by many Medicare recipients until they actually require long-term care. A basic issue is simply defining the types of services, and which of these services should be included in long-term care. One typical definition, provided by the Medicare administration on their Web site, is that long-term care includes medical and non-medical care to those who have a chronic illness or disability. Long-term care can also help meet health or personal needs. Often, long-term care assists people with needs for support services such as activities of daily living (dressing, bathing, and using the bathroom). Long-term care does not have to be provided in a nursing home; it can also be provided at home, in the community, or more recently, in an assisted living setting. Medicare does cover some nursing home and home care, and what care is actually covered now is different than when Medicare legislation was first passed in 1965. However, in general, Medicare does not cover routine nursing home care unless it is related to a recent hospitalization or other urgent medical treatment. Those types of needs are covered under Part A of Medicare and are often known as extended care services. Most long-term care helps people with support services such as activities of daily living (dressing, bathing, using the bathroom, and feeding oneself). These are not covered by Medicare which considers these types of services custodial care.

Medicare will pay for 100 days of nursing home care for people with a prior hospital stay who need skilled nursing care or rehabilitative therapy. Generally, Medicare will pay the full costs of care for the first 20 days of a nursing home stay, but after that period, Medicare beneficiaries have a substantial copayment (over $125 a day). Coverage for home health care by Medicare is also limited to people with skilled care needs. To receive home health care, a person must be homebound, need intermittent skilled nursing or other therapy services, and be under the care of a physician to prescribe a plan of home care. Home health aide services such as assistance with dressing, transferring, and toileting can be provided if people also have skilled care needs. The home health benefit is not tied to a recent hospitalization, there is no limit on the number of days of care or home visits a person can receive, and there is also no cost-sharing requirement. In 2004, about 6 percent of Medicare beneficiaries received home health services, averaging 31 home health visits. In 2005, Medicare spent about 4 percent of its funds on home health care and 6 percent on nursing home care (Medicare and Long Term Care Fact Sheet, 2007). By 2008, these figures were about equal, 5 percent on nursing home care and 4 percent on home health care (The Long-term Outlook for Medicare, Medicaid, and Total Health Care Spending, 2008).

Not all elderly will use long-term care services in their lifetime. Medicare estimates that currently about nine million elderly over the age of 65 will need long-term care and that the figure could grow to 12 million by 2020. Most of this care will not be provided in an institutional setting, but at home by family and friends. Estimates are that people who reach age 65 will likely have a 40 percent chance of entering a nursing home in the future, with about 10 percent of the people who enter a nursing home residing there five years or more (Culyer and Newhouse, 2000; Kemper and Murtaugh, 1991).

People can buy private long-term care insurance, but it is often quite expensive which reflects the small number of those who buy such policies at present. There are several limitations on current insurance policies. As

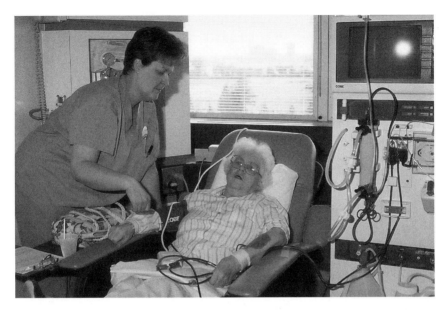

An elderly woman receives medical treatment in a hospital. Medicare offers hospital coverage, but little in the way of long-term care coverage. (Corel)

mentioned, they are generally expensive, usually more than $1,000 a month for a couple, so this puts such policies out of the range of many as they prepare for retirement in their late 50's and 60's. Financial experts often point out that, if a person is to buy such a policy, it is very important to understand how much care is provided and how the care is priced. In the past, some policies set a dollar amount per day which may have sounded reasonable at the time the policy was issued (for example, to someone 60 years old), but ended being an amount that was far below the current costs of a day of nursing home care for someone in their mid-80s, twenty-five years after the policy was issued. Some policies people currently try to use were written before assisted living options were created, and thus, will only cover nursing home care. It is difficult to anticipate changes in the ways long-term care will be provided in the future and to be sure that policies are written broadly enough to cover all options. These limitations, along with the high cost of the policies and the confusion that people have about whether this coverage is part of Medicare, have tended to curb public interest in long-term care coverage.

MEDICAID AS A SOURCE OF LONG-TERM CARE COVERAGE

Medicaid is a government program that has become an important provider of nursing home care (and, in many states, home-based care as well). In contrast to Medicare, which most elderly in the United States receive,

Medicaid is a means-tested program and most elderly do not initially qualify. In all states, these means tests both include an income limit and also asset tests for people to qualify. The way in which the program ends up paying for long-term care services for many people is through what has often been called a "spend-down" procedure. When nursing home care is required, most people initially pay for the expenses using their private assets. As these personal resources are exhausted, they then check on their eligibility for Medicaid to assume the remaining costs of long-term care. People can become eligible because their medical costs are so high that they are determined to be "medically needy" even though their income is above the general level of eligibility for Medicaid.

One past issue was that the house in which a spouse lived would be counted as an asset: thus, the other spouse needing nursing home care was declared ineligible for Medicaid unless the house was sold. This sometimes prompted the couple to divorce so that the spouse in poor health could qualify for Medicaid while the other spouse could remain in the house in which they had often lived for many years. Now, a house in which a spouse is living does not count against the other spouse as an asset, within some limits. In 1988, Congress enacted provisions to prevent what became known as "spousal impoverishment," which left the spouse still living at home in the community with little or no income or resources. These provisions help ensure that community spouses are also able to live out their lives with independence and dignity. The spousal impoverishment provision applies when one member of a couple enters a nursing facility and is expected to be there for over thirty days. An assessment of the couples' resources will be made when they apply for Medicaid, but the home, household goods, automobile, and burial funds are not included in the couple's combined resources. Giving resources to family or friends can render a person ineligible for Medicaid or a person may be assessed a penalty if the state discovers that assets were given away too close to the need for long-term care. These provisions are to make sure that the people who receive Medicaid need the program to pay for long-term care, and not simply to preserve assets for their heirs.

The increased costs of long-term care and the rising number of elderly needing such care have modified Medicaid expenditures in many states so that long-term care spending is now a very important part of the Medicaid burden. This recent trend is not new as Medicaid spending for long-term care increased 9.3 percent from fiscal year 1996 to fiscal year 1997—the highest rate of growth in long-term care spending since fiscal year 1992 (Coleman, 1999). Home care spending as a percentage of total Medicaid long-term care spending more than doubled from 1987 to 1997, from 10.8 percent to 24 percent (Coleman, 1999). By 2008, averaging across states, and even considering that the elderly and disabled make up about one-quarter of Medicaid's enrollees, the former account for two-thirds of the program's spending. This is one of the ways in which Medicaid has now, in terms of expenditures, become an important program for health coverage of the elderly. Overall, about one-third of Medicaid's spending in fiscal year 2008 was for long-term care, which includes nursing home services, home health care, and other medical and social services for people whose disabilities prevent them from living independently (The Long-term Outlook for Medicare, Medicaid, and Total Health Care Spending, 2008).

Most experts do not expect the need for long-term care services, especially near the end of life, to decline in coming decades as the U.S. population is aging, led by the baby boomers who will be reaching retirement ages in the next decades. How to pay for the services for a larger number of recipients will remain an issue, both for individual beneficiaries of Medicare and for government programs overall. In the new health reform legislation of the Obama administration, there are some changes that relate to home- and community-based services in Medicare. There will be an elimination of Part D (drug) cost-sharing for full-benefit, dual-eligible beneficiaries receiving home- and community-based services. It is too soon to understand the full impact of the legislation, but this section will briefly summarize a number of other changes, as mentioned by leading gerontology professional associations, such as the Gerontological Society of America. The legislation will modify the spousal impoverishment laws and order states to include spousal impoverishment protections in their waiver programs. This will provide spouses of all HCBS (Home and Community Based Services) waiver participants, including those who qualify as medically needy, with all available protections. These new provisions will sunset (disappear) after five years, as the legislation will expect other changes to begin to occur. The 2010 health reform bill will also extend some rebalancing demonstration programs through 2016 to encourage states to transition Medicare-enrolled individuals from nursing homes to communities.

A new program will be created, the Community First Choice Option, to help provide community-based attendant support and services to individuals with disabilities who are Medicaid-eligible and who require an institutional level of care. States that choose the Community First Choice Option will be eligible for an enhanced federal match rate. Included with this program is required data collection to help determine how states currently are providing home- and community-based services, the cost of those services, and whether states currently offer individuals with disabilities, who otherwise qualify for institutional care under Medicaid, the choice to instead receive home- and community-based services, as required by the U.S. Supreme Court decision, *Olmstead v. L.C.* in 1999.

A new national long-term care insurance program will be created though voluntary payroll deductions and will provide a cash benefit to individuals who need help in basic activities of daily living to help them purchase community living assistance and support. How this will apply to current Medicare beneficiaries is not clear from the legislation. One goal of the new program will be to help reduce Medicare deficits by $57.8 billion over the next 10 years due to the payment of premiums by enrollees (the voluntary payroll deductions). A national clearinghouse on long-term care information will be created and all of these changes should result in federal and state Medicaid savings of $4.4 billion.

There will also be new measures for care coordination that will include the creation of an Independence at Home demonstration program to provide high-need Medicare beneficiaries with primary care services in their homes and allow participating teams of health professionals to share in any savings if they reduce preventable hospitalizations, prevent hospital readmissions, improve health outcomes and the efficiency of care, reduce the cost of health care services, and achieve patient satisfaction. There will also be an Innovation Center at the Centers for Medicare and Medicaid Services that will be created to look for different Medicare and Medicaid payment structures that could foster patient-centered care and care coordination across treatment settings and slow cost growth. The impact of all these new programs and approaches will be closely watched in the coming years. While these programs include goals of saving money and allowing states to benefit from those savings, given the current economic problems and the funding crisis in many states, the issue of using Medicaid-matching funds to pay for some of these new care services will also continue to be a serious concern.

MEDICARE AND THE DEMOGRAPHIC-BASED FUNDING CRISIS

One statistic repeated often in the popular media is that the Medicare program is "going broke" and will eventually run out of funds in the near future. The idea that there was a crisis in Medicare funding was the focus of much discussion, especially beginning in the 1990s, although there were also funding crises during 1969–1972 and 1983–1984. But prior to the mid-1990s' crisis, Democrats and Republicans generally were in agreement about how to respond to shortfalls in Medicare funding, decisions were made by policymakers, not by politicians, and issues were generally handled in a bipartisan manner (Oberlander, 2003). The shift from bipartisanship to politically-based debates occurred with the 1995 Medicare-funding crisis. At that time, Congressional Republicans presented a Medicare reform package that was based upon projections of insolvency of the program in 2002. As part of the Congressional debate, Republican leadership argued that Medicare first faced a short-term financial crisis, and second, a longer-term problem in which they projected that unless major changes were implemented, the program would be bankrupt by 2010. This coincided with the year the baby-boomer generation would begin to retire and start to double the number of Medicare beneficiaries over the next two decades. The issue of Medicare trust fund shortfalls transformed from objective events that needed discussion and response into political events of a subjective nature. Solutions began to reflect partisan political party alignments and basic ideology.

To understand this new direction, a review of the different funding mechanisms for Medicare will be discussed in this section. As previously mentioned, Part A for hospital care is funded through matching payroll taxes from workers and employers and has the concept of a trust fund. Physician funding (Part B) and the more recently added drug coverage (Part D) rely upon beneficiary premiums and matching general revenues from the federal government. Much of the confusion about Medicare running out of funds stems from the Part A funding provisions, which mirrors the way Social Security was funded. Drawing upon a social insurance model, the original notion of this funding approach for Social Security was to provide a moral claim on future benefits and separate the benefits from welfare-based, means-tested programs. The initial idea was that Part A of Medicare would also be self-supporting as is Social Security.

In reality, that assumption has never really been true for Medicare. Two of the measures that actuaries of Medicare calculate to see how the program is holding up financially are: 1) a projection of the number of years until the Medicare hospitalization trust fund will be exhausted, and 2) the size of the long-term deficit in the hospitalization insurance trust fund. Medicare's long-range actuarial balance has been negative almost from the beginning of the program. This means that the revenues have been projected as not being sufficient to cover costs for the upcoming twenty-five year period. Oberlander (2003) argues that for 26 of the past 30 years of the operation of Medicare, there has been a long-range trust fund deficit and there was no positive actuarial balance from 1974 to 1994. In the discussions within the public arena, there are some links between number of years of trust fund exhaustion and the perception of Medicare financial crises. Oberlander (2003) reports that there were three periods in which the estimated time until trust fund exhaustion was less than seven years: 1969–1972, 1982–1984, and 1993–1995.

One problem is that actuarial computations about Social Security are much simpler than for Medicare, because those projections are based only upon demographic trends and future benefits owed to contributing workers. To project Medicare costs, not only are demographics and enrollment numbers involved, but also estimates of future rates of utilization of health care services, the costs of those services, the changes in patterns of care due to changes in technology, and even trends in disability and chronic disease patterns. Thus, these factors make the projection process more complicated, less straightforward, and more difficult for Medicare.

However, these projections, to some extent, drive the public's and policy makers' assessments of how serious the financial problems are for Medicare. If Medicare had been funded just through general revenues and the assets of Part A were not, in some ways, maintained in a separate account, then the program's finances could not be used up in the same way as are the finances for Social Security. Due to the difficulty of forecasting, actuarial estimates in Medicare have not been a source of stabilization for Medicare, but actually lead to trust fund crises which are partially real and partially created situations. Some experts argue that financing Medicare Part A by general revenues rather than by the trust fund would eliminate this problem (Oberlander, 2003). In the past 30 years, there has been political discussion about this proposed financing, but policy experts, as well as some lawmakers, fear that the efforts for financial discipline in the program would be reduced. For the Part B physician payments and the newer Part D drug programs, the costs are met mostly from revenues from beneficiaries and sometimes, from general tax revenues. Here the concern is partially that costs will increase so much that the expense of being in the program begin to decrease the usable incomes of the elderly.

Still, the most recent estimates of the financial future for Medicare are not encouraging. Medicare, which serves more than 43 million elderly and disabled people, is in worse shape than Social Security and the Board of Trustees have said the Medicare hospital insurance trust fund is projected to be insolvent by 2019 (Lee, 2007). There is one projection that by 2012, Medicare and Social Security combined could consume 10 percent of federal income tax revenue, and increase to 26 percent by 2020 (Lee, 2007). Political leaders, both within Congress and the President, would be forced to make a decision whether to increase taxes, reduce Medicare (and Social Security) benefits, or to do both. Medicare Trustees have warned that based on new projections, money from general revenues could exceed 45 percent of projected Medicare expenditures in two consecutive years, 2012 and 2013. Currently, 42 percent of Medicare outlays are from general revenue. Medicare's financial problems have been increased by the passage of the Part D drug benefit, which cost the government about $30 billion in 2006 (Lee, 2007).

When U.S. population estimates are carefully analyzed, the number of people projected to be on Medicare will become quite large. In the 2000 U.S. census, the Medicare-eligible population totaled 35.1 million. Based upon that same census data, the estimates are that by 2030 the Medicare-eligible population is projected to increase to 69.7 million, and by 2050 to 81.9 million (U.S. Census Bureau, 2000). Even if health care costs did not continue to increase and new, more expensive technologies were not developed and implemented, the cost of Medicare is projected to increase. Given expectations of improved health and longevity, it is not unreasonable to project even a larger number of people on Medicare and even

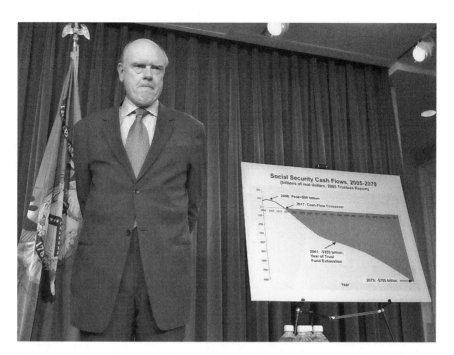

Treasury Secretary John Snow, who is also chairman of the board of trustees for Social Security and Medicare, stands by a chart detailing future Social Security cash flows during a news conference at the Treasury Department, March 23, 2005. The trust fund for Social Security will go broke in 2041—a year earlier than previously estimated—the trustees reported. Trustees also said that Medicare, the giant health care program for the elderly and disabled, faces insolvency in 2020. Obama health reforms include some ways to cut costs in Medicare and thus, improve the financial picture for Medicare in the future. (AP Photo/Charles Dharapak)

higher medical costs. Perhaps, some costs might be lowered if recipients live longer but are healthier, but health care costs generally rise with aging, ending with the often very high costs found in a person's last decade of life. Some experts, however, do offer a more positive outlook on future Medicare costs. Reinhardt (2003), a well-known health economist, argues that while in any given year per capita health spending for people age 65 or older tends to average three to five times more than that for younger Americans, the aging of the population is too gradual a process to rank as a major cost driver in health care. This is a more optimistic outlook on future Medicare costs.

In the past decade, policy analysts have examined a variety of ways to create real savings in the Medicare program. Some argue that real savings to Medicare can occur within a five-year time frame and with only modest changes in providers' behaviors (Fisher et al., 2009). The trick, these experts argue, is to slow spending growth while improving quality of care. Some believe that this can be accomplished by making care more integrated and efficient and fostering greater accountability for quality and costs through performance measurement (Fisher et al., 2009; Crosson, 2009). Other experts point out that the public must be convinced that less care can be positive and not be considered "rationing" and that receiving more care does not necessarily mean receiving better-quality care (Rother, 2009). Still others point out that the system to hold down physician costs in Medicare has been overridden by Congress in every year since 2003 and that achieving cost control means readdressing how physicians are paid and how their payments are determined (Laugesen, 2009).

The new health reform legislation of the Obama administration, through the spending cuts in the Medicare Advantage plan, does anticipate some improvement in the Medicare trust fund. The provisions for equalizing payments between Advantage plans and traditional Medicare are based upon a recommendation by the non-partisan Medicare Payment Advisory Commission (MedPAC), and are supported by advocates for Medicare beneficiaries such as the Center for Medicare Advocacy. One purpose of these provisions is to extend the life of the Medicare Trust Fund which, without some intervention, is now projected to be depleted in 2017. These Medicare Advantage cuts will result in approximately $118 billion in savings. In addition, other parts of the new health reform legislation will bring in about $500 billion in savings over the next 10 years from the previously expected future growth of Medicare. Estimates indicate this should extend the life of the program for nine or so more years, relieving some pressure to immediately cut benefits or to increase premiums. However, all of these figures are projections and preliminary estimates, and thus could change over time.

The future of Medicare payments and Medicare funding is not clear at this time. Some experts point out that payment reform alone cannot be expected to transform health care delivery, whether looking at just the Medicare program or at all of health care (Kahn, 2009). Issues of the future of Medicare clearly relate to issues of overall health care reform, and to reform in Medicare specifically, which is the topic of the last section of this chapter.

MEDICARE AND HEALTH CARE REFORM

This book has reviewed a number of problems and concerns with the Medicare program. During the period 2009–2010, many policy experts believed that health care reform might make Medicare, as a separate program with all its specific details, a program of the past in the United States. Other experts thought that Medicare might be expanded to cover more people and broader age groups and thus, become the basis for a public option in health care reform. Instead, neither prediction has occurred. Health care reform has become health insurance reform, with less focus on the Medicare program. There are real issues about payment in Medicare and how to reform Medicare that are not being addressed this year, although the new Obama legislation does create some "fixes" for drug payments, some attempts to save money and extend the life of the Medicare Trust Funds, and a number of approaches to look at issues related to long-term care and home- and community-based services. To the extent that the reform debate has focused on Medicare, however, more of the discussion has been about how to find savings within the program to help pay for health insurance for other age groups. At times, this has made seniors very concerned about Medicare being damaged and their options decreased. Certainly, higher-income individuals will pay more in the future for their Part B and Part D benefits. In addition, current workers will pay a higher tax on wages beginning in 2013 and there will be other new Medicare taxes for individuals that earn more than $200,000 a year or for couples that jointly earn more than $250,000 a year. There will also be a tax on unearned income such as dividends and interest. These additional taxes will help to fund health care reform overall, but it is not clear how they will relate to Medicare-specific funds, and some experts believe that differences between separate funds and programs may diminish as additional modifications are likely to be made to the health reform provisions enacted in 2010. As when Medicare was first enacted in 1965, new legislation may have yet unexpected impacts, and lead to changes that are not possible to predict at this point in time.

References and Resources

Annotated Primary Source Documents

MEDICARE LEGISLATION, TITLE XVIII OF THE SOCIAL SECURITY LEGISLATION

This section of the book includes selected portions of the legislation, with a focus upon more general parts and the basic parts of most interest for people conducting more general research on Medicare. Included below are selections from the general introductory material and the most relevant portions of the legislation on Parts A, B, C, and D. Excluded from the general introductory material are section 1805—Medicare Payment Advisory Commission, and Section 1807—Chronic Care Improvements. Excluded from Part A are section 1814 on Conditions and Limitations on Payments for Services, section 1819 on requirements for, and assuring quality of care in skilled nursing facilities, section 1820 on rural hospital flexibility program, and section 1821 conditions for coverage of religious nonmedical health care institutional services. Excluded from Part B are all parts of section 1833, Payments of Benefits except sections 1, 2, and 3, section 1824 on special payment rules for particular items of service, section 1837 on enrollment periods, section 1838 on coverage period, section 1840 on payment of premiums, section 1841 on federal supplementary medical insurance trust fund, section 1842 on provisions relating to administration of Part B, section 1844 on appropriations to cover government contribution and contingency reserve, the repealed section 1845, section 1846 on intermediate sanctions for providers or suppliers of clinical laboratory drug tests, and section 1847 on competitive acquisitions of certain items and services including parts a and b on use of average sales price payment methodology and competitive acquisition of outpatient drugs and biologicals. For Part B, section 1848 on payments for physician services, only part 1 is included. For Part C, only section 1851 is included.

Since only a small subset of Medicare recipients elect Medicare + Choice, the rest of the details are not included. This includes sections 1852 through 1859 that focus on benefits and beneficiary protections, payments to Medicare + Choice organizations, premiums and premium amounts, organizations and financial requirements, establishment of standards, contracts and special rules and definitions. For Part D, the Voluntary Prescription Drug Benefit Program, subpart 1 on Part D, Eligible Individuals and Prescription Drug Benefits, sections 1860D— Eligible Individuals and the prescription drug program is included as is section 1860D—2, prescription drug benefits. The rest of 1860D section 3, Access to a choice of qualified prescription drug coverage and section 4, Beneficiary protections for qualified prescription drug coverage are not included. Also excluded are all of Subpart 2—Prescription Drug Plans; PDP Sponsors; Financing and Subpart 3—Application to Medicare Advantage Program and Treatment of Employer-Sponsored Programs and Other Prescription Drug Plans, and Subpart 4—Medicare Prescription Drug Discount Card and Transitional Assistance Program and Subpart 5—Definitions and Miscellaneous Provisions. Part E the final material on miscellaneous provisions is not included.

Prohibition against Any Federal Interference

Sec. 1801. [42 U.S.C. 1395] Nothing in this title shall be construed to authorize any Federal officer or employee to exercise any supervision or control over the practice of medicine or the manner in which medical services are provided, or over the selection, tenure, or compensation of any officer or employee of any institution, agency, or person providing health services; or to exercise any supervision or control over the administration or operation of any such institution, agency, or person.

Free Choice by Patient Guaranteed

Sec. 1802. [42 U.S.C. 1395a]

(a) Basic freedom of choice.—Any individual entitled to insurance benefits under this title may obtain health services from any institution, agency, or person qualified to participate under this title if such institution, agency, or person undertakes to provide him such services.

(b) Use of Private Contracts by Medicare Beneficiaries.—

    (1) In general.—Subject to the provisions of this subsection, nothing in this title shall prohibit a physician or practitioner from entering into a private contract with a medicare beneficiary for any item or service—

    (A) for which no claim for payment is to be submitted under this title, and

    (B) for which the physician or practitioner receives—

        (i) no reimbursement under this title directly or on a capitated basis, and

        (ii) receives no amount for such item or service from an organization which receives reimbursement for such item or service under this title directly or on a capitated basis.

    (2) Beneficiary protections.—

    (A) In general.—Paragraph (1) shall not apply to any contract unless—

        (i) the contract is in writing and is signed by the medicare beneficiary before any item or service is provided pursuant to the contract;

        (ii) the contract contains the items described in subparagraph (B); and

        (iii) the contract is not entered into at a time when the medicare beneficiary is facing an emergency or urgent health care situation.

(B) Items required to be included in contract.—Any contract to provide items and services to which paragraph (1) applies shall clearly indicate to the medicare beneficiary that by signing such contract the beneficiary—

    (i) agrees not to submit a claim (or to request that the physician or practitioner submit a claim) under this title for such items or services even if such items or services are otherwise covered by this title;

    (ii) agrees to be responsible, whether through insurance or otherwise, for payment of such items or services and understands that no reimbursement will be provided under this title for such items or services;

    (iii) acknowledges that no limits under this title (including the limits under section 1848(g)) apply to amounts that may be charged for such items or services;

    (iv) acknowledges that Medigap plans under section 1882 do not, and other supplemental insurance plans may elect not to, make payments for such items and services because payment is not made under this title; and

    (v) acknowledges that the medicare beneficiary has the right to have such items or services provided by other physicians or practitioners for whom payment would be made under this title.

Such contract shall also clearly indicate whether the physician or practitioner is excluded from participation under the medicare program under section 1128.

(3) Physician or practitioner requirements.—

    (A) In general.—Paragraph (1) shall not apply to any contract entered into by a physician or practitioner unless an affidavit described in subparagraph (B) is in effect during the period any item or service is to be provided pursuant to the contract.

    (B) Affidavit.—An affidavit is described in this subparagraph if—

        (i) the affidavit identifies the physician or practitioner and is in writing and is signed by the physician or practitioner;

        (ii) the affidavit provides that the physician or practitioner will not submit any claim under this title for any item or service provided to any medicare beneficiary (and will not receive any reimbursement or amount described in paragraph (1)(B) for any such item or service) during the 2-year period beginning on the date the affidavit is signed; and

        (iii) a copy of the affidavit is filed with the Secretary no later than 10 days after the first contract to which such affidavit applies is entered into.

    (C) Enforcement.—If a physician or practitioner signing an affidavit under subparagraph (B) knowingly and willfully submits a claim under this title for any item or service provided during the 2-year period described in subparagraph (B)(ii) (or receives any reimbursement or amount described in paragraph (1)(B) for any such item or service) with respect to such affidavit—

    (i) this subsection shall not apply with respect to any items and services provided by the physician or practitioner pursuant to any contract on and after the date of such submission and before the end of such period; and

    (ii) no payment shall be made under this title for any item or service furnished by the physician or practitioner during the period described in clause (i) (and no reimbursement or payment of any amount described in paragraph (1)(B) shall be made for any such item or service).

(4) Limitation on actual charge and claim submission requirement not applicable.—Section 1848(g) shall not apply with respect to any item or service provided to a medicare beneficiary under a contract described in paragraph (1).

(5) Definitions.—In this subsection:

    (A) Medicare beneficiary.—The term "medicare beneficiary" means an individual who is entitled to benefits under part A or enrolled under part B.

    (B) Physician.—The term "physician" has the meaning given such term by paragraphs (1), (2), (3), and (4) of section 1861(r).

    (C) Practitioner.—The term "practitioner" has the meaning given such term by section 1842(b)(18)(C).

Option to Individuals to Obtain Other Health Insurance Protection

Sec. 1803. [42 U.S.C. 1395b] Nothing contained in this title shall be construed to preclude any State from providing, or any individual from purchasing or otherwise securing, protection against the cost of any health services.

Notice of Medicare Benefits: Medicare and Medigap Information[3]

Sec. 1804. [42 U.S.C. 1395b-2]

(a) The Secretary shall prepare (in consultation with groups representing the elderly and with health insurers) and provide for distribution of a notice containing—

(1) a clear, simple explanation of the benefits available under this title and the major categories of health care for which benefits are not available under this title,

(2) the limitations on payment (including deductibles and coinsurance amounts) that are imposed under this title, and

(3) a description of the limited benefits for long-term care services available under this title and generally available under State plans approved under title XIX.

Such notice shall be mailed annually to individuals entitled to benefits under part A or part B of this title and when an individual applies for benefits under part A or enrolls under part B.

(b) The Secretary shall provide information via a toll-free telephone number on the programs under this title. The Secretary shall provide, through the toll-free telephone number 1-800-MEDICARE, for a means by which individuals seeking information about, or assistance with, such programs who phone such toll-free number are transferred (without charge) to appropriate entities for the provision of such information or assistance. Such toll-free number shall be the toll-free number listed for general information and assistance in the annual notice under subsection (a) instead of the listing of numbers of individual contractors.[4]

(c) The notice provided under subsection (a) shall include—

(1) a statement which indicates that because errors do occur and because medicare fraud, waste, and abuse is a significant problem, beneficiaries should carefully check any explanation of benefits or itemized statement furnished pursuant to section 1806 for accuracy and report any errors or questionable charges by calling the toll-free phone number described in paragraph (4);

(2) a statement of the beneficiary's right to request an itemized statement for medicare items and services (as provided in section 1806(b));

(3) a description of the program to collect information on medicare fraud and abuse established under section 203(b) of the Health Insurance Portability and Accountability Act of 1996[5]; and

(4) a toll-free telephone number maintained by the Inspector General in the Department of Health and Human Services for the receipt of complaints and information about waste, fraud, and abuse in the provision or billing of services under this title.

Explanation of Medicare Benefits[10]

Sec. 1806. [42 U.S.C. 1395b–7]

(a) In General.—The Secretary shall furnish to each individual for whom payment has been made under this title (or would be made without regard to any deductible) a statement which—

(1) lists the item or service for which payment has been made and the amount of such payment for each item or service; and

(2) includes a notice of the individual's right to request an itemized statement (as provided in subsection (b)).

(b) Request for itemized statement for medicare items and services.—

(1) In general.—An individual may submit a written request to any physician, provider, supplier, or any other person (including an organization, agency, or other entity) for an itemized statement for any item or service provided to such individual by such person with respect to which payment has been made under this title.

(2) 30-day period to furnish statement.—

(A) In general.—Not later than 30 days after the date on which a request under paragraph (1) has been made, a person described in such paragraph shall furnish an itemized statement describing each item or service provided to the individual requesting the itemized statement.

(B) Penalty.—Whoever knowingly fails to furnish an itemized statement in accordance with subparagraph (A) shall be subject to a civil money penalty of not more than $100 for each such failure. Such penalty shall be imposed and collected in the same manner as civil money penalties under subsection (a) of section 1128A are imposed and collected under that section.

(3) Review of itemized statement.—

(A) In general.—Not later than 90 days after the receipt of an itemized statement furnished under paragraph (1), an individual may submit a written request for a review of the itemized statement to the Secretary.

(B) Specific allegations.—A request for a review of the itemized statement shall identify—

(i) specific items or services that the individual believes were not provided as claimed, or

(ii) any other billing irregularity (including duplicate billing).

(4) Findings of secretary.—The Secretary shall, with respect to each written request submitted under paragraph (3), determine whether the itemized statement identifies specific items or services that were not provided as claimed or any other billing irregularity (including duplicate billing) that has resulted in unnecessary payments under this title.

(5) Recovery of amounts.—The Secretary shall take all appropriate measures to recover amounts unnecessarily paid under this title with respect to a statement described in paragraph (4).

Provisions Relating to Administration

Sec. 1808. [42 U.S.C. 1395b–9]

(a) Coordinated Administration of Medicare Prescription Drug and Medicare Advantage Programs.—

(1) In general.—There is within the Centers for Medicare and Medicaid Services a center to carry out the duties described in paragraph (3).

(2) Director.—Such center shall be headed by a director who shall report directly to the Administrator of the Centers for Medicare and Medicaid Services.

(3) Duties.—The duties described in this paragraph are the following:

(A) The administration of parts C and D.

(B) The provision of notice and information under section 1804.

(C) Such other duties as the Secretary may specify.

(4) Deadline.—The Secretary shall ensure that the center is carrying out the duties described in paragraph (3) by not later than January 1, 2008.

(b) Employment Of Management Staff.—

(1) In general.—The Secretary may employ, within the Centers for Medicare and Medicaid Services, such individuals as management staff as the Secretary determines to be appropriate. With respect to the administration of parts C and D, such individuals shall include individuals with private sector expertise in negotiations with health benefits plans.

(2) Eligibility.—To be eligible for employment under paragraph (1) an individual shall be required to have demonstrated, by their education and experience (either in the public or private sector), superior expertise in at least one of the following areas:

(A) The review, negotiation, and administration of health care contracts.

(B) The design of health care benefit plans.

(C) Actuarial sciences.

(D) Compliance with health plan contracts.

(E) Consumer education and decision making.

(F) Any other area specified by the Secretary that requires specialized management or other expertise.

(3) Rates of payment.—

(A) Performance-related pay.—Subject to subparagraph (B), the Secretary shall establish the rate of pay for an individual employed under paragraph (1). Such rate shall take into account expertise, experience, and performance.

(B) Limitation.—In no case may the rate of compensation determined under subparagraph (A) exceed the highest rate of basic pay for the Senior Executive Service under section 5382(b) of title 5, United States Code.

(c) Medicare Beneficiary Ombudsman.—

(1) In general.—The Secretary shall appoint within the Department of Health and Human Services a Medicare Beneficiary Ombudsman who shall have expertise and experience in the fields of health care and education of (and assistance to) individuals entitled to benefits under this title.

(2) Duties.—The Medicare Beneficiary Ombudsman shall—

(A) receive complaints, grievances, and requests for information submitted by individuals entitled to benefits under part A or enrolled under part B, or both, with respect to any aspect of the medicare program;

(B) provide assistance with respect to complaints, grievances, and requests referred to in subparagraph (A), including—

(i) assistance in collecting relevant information for such individuals, to seek an appeal of a decision or determination made by a fiscal intermediary, carrier, MA organization, or the Secretary

(ii) assistance to such individuals with any problems arising from disenrollment from an MA plan under part C; and

(iii) assistance to such individuals in presenting information under section 1839(i)(4)(C) (relating to income-related premium adjustment); and

(C) submit annual reports to Congress and the Secretary that describe the activities of the Office and that include such recommendations for improvement in the administration of this title as the Ombudsman determines appropriate. The Ombudsman shall not serve as an advocate for any increases in payments or new coverage of services, but may identify issues and problems in payment or coverage policies.

(3) Working with health insurance counseling programs.—To the extent possible, the Ombudsman shall work with health insurance counseling programs (receiving funding under section 4360 of Omnibus Budget Reconciliation Act of 1990) to facilitate the provision of information to individuals entitled to benefits under part A or enrolled under part B, or both regarding MA plans and changes to those plans. Nothing in this paragraph shall preclude further collaboration between the Ombudsman and such programs.

Addressing Health Care Disparities[12]

Sec. 1809. [42 U.S.C. 1395b-10]

(a) Evaluating Data Collection Approaches.—The Secretary shall evaluate approaches for the collection of data under this title, to be performed in conjunction with existing quality reporting requirements and programs under this title, that allow for the ongoing, accurate, and timely collection and evaluation of data on disparities in health care services and performance on the basis of race, ethnicity, and gender. In conducting such evaluation, the Secretary shall consider the following objectives:

(1) Protecting patient privacy.

(2) Minimizing the administrative burdens of data collection and reporting on providers and health plans participating under this title.

(3) Improving Medicare program data on race, ethnicity, and gender.

(b) Reports to Congress.—

(1) Report on evaluation.—Not later than 18 months after the date of the enactment of this section, the Secretary shall submit to Congress a report on the evaluation conducted under subsection (a). Such report shall, taking into consideration the results of such evaluation—

(A) identify approaches (including defining methodologies) for identifying and collecting and evaluating data on health care disparities on the basis of race, ethnicity, and gender for the original Medicare fee-for-service program under parts A and B, the Medicare Advantage program under part C, and the Medicare prescription drug program under part D; and

(B) include recommendations on the most effective strategies and approaches to reporting HEDIS quality measures as required under section 1852(e)(3) and other nationally recognized quality performance measures, as appropriate, on the basis of race, ethnicity, and gender.

(2) Reports on data analyses.—Not later than 4 years after the date of the enactment of this section, and 4 years thereafter, the Secretary shall submit to Congress a report that includes recommendations for improving the identification of health care disparities for Medicare beneficiaries based on analyses of the data collected under subsection (c).

(c) Implementing Effective Approaches.—Not later than 24 months after the date of the enactment of this section, the Secretary shall implement the approaches identified in the report submitted under subsection (b)(1) for the ongoing, accurate, and timely collection and evaluation of data on health care disparities on the basis of race, ethnicity, and gender.

Part A—Hospital Insurance Benefits for the Aged and Disabled[13]

Description of Program

Sec. 1811. [42 U.S.C. 1395c] The insurance program for which entitlement is established by sections 226 and 226A provides basic protection against the costs of hospital, related post-hospital, home health services, and hospice care in accordance with this part for (1) individuals who are age 65 or over and are eligible for retirement benefits under title II of this Act (or would be eligible for such benefits if certain government employment were covered employment under such title) or under the railroad retirement system, (2) individuals under age 65 who have been entitled for not less than 24 months to benefits under title II of this Act (or would have been so entitled to such benefits if certain government employment were covered employment under such title) or under the railroad retirement system on the basis of a disability, and (3) certain individuals who do not meet the conditions specified in either clause (1) or (2) but who are medically determined to have end stage renal disease.

Scope of Benefits

Sec. 1812. [42 U.S.C. 1395d]

(a) The benefits provided to an individual by the insurance program under this part shall consist of entitlement to have payment made on his behalf or, in the case of payments referred to in section 1814(d)(2) to him (subject to the provisions of this part) for—

  (1) inpatient hospital services or inpatient critical access hospital services for up to 150 days during any spell of illness minus 1 day for each day of such services in excess of 90 received during any preceding spell of illness (if such individual was entitled to have payment for such services made under this part unless he specifies in accordance with regulations of the Secretary that he does not desire to have such payment made);

  (2)(A) post-hospital extended care services for up to 100 days during any spell of illness, and (B) to the extent provided in subsection (f), extended care services that are not post-hospital extended care services;

  (3) in the case of individuals not enrolled in part B, home health services, and for individuals so enrolled, post-institutional home health services furnished during a home health spell of illness for up to 100 visits during such spell of illness;

  (4) in lieu of certain other benefits, hospice care with respect to the individual during up to two periods of 90 days each and an unlimited number of subsequent periods of 60 days each with respect to which the individual makes an election under subsection (d)(1); and

  (5) for individuals who are terminally ill, have not made an election under subsection (d)(1), and have not previously received services under this paragraph, services that are furnished by a physician (as defined in section 1861(r)(1)) who is either the medical director or an employee of a hospice program and that—

(A) consist of—

    (i) an evaluation of the individual's need for pain and symptom management, including the individual's need for hospice care; and

    (ii) counseling the individual with respect to hospice care and other care options; and

(B) may include advising the individual regarding advanced care planning.

(b) Payment under this part for services furnished an individual during a spell of illness may not (subject to subsection (c)) be made for—

    (1) inpatient hospital services furnished to him during such spell after such services have been furnished to him for 150 days during such spell minus 1 day for each day of inpatient hospital services in excess of 90 received during any preceding spell of illness (if such individual was entitled to have payment for such services made under this part unless he specifies in accordance with regulations of the Secretary that he does not desire to have such payment made);

    (2) post-hospital extended care services furnished to him during such spell after such services have been furnished to him for 100 days during such spell; or

    (3) inpatient psychiatric hospital services furnished to him after such services have been furnished to him for a total of 190 days during his lifetime.

Payment under this part for post-institutional home health services furnished an individual during a home health spell of illness may not be made for such services beginning after such services have been furnished for a total of 100 visits during such spell

(c) If an individual is an inpatient of a psychiatric hospital on the first day of the first month for which he is entitled to benefits under this part, the days on which he was an inpatient of such a hospital in the 150-day period immediately before such first day shall be included in determining the number of days limit under subsection (b)(1) insofar as such limit applies to (1) inpatient psychiatric hospital services, or (2) inpatient hospital services for an individual who is an inpatient primarily for the diagnosis or treatment of mental illness (but shall not be included in determining such number of days limit insofar as it applies to other inpatient hospital services or in determining the 190-day limit under subsection (b)(3).

(d)(1) Payment under this part may be made for hospice care provided with respect to an individual only during two periods of 90 days each and an unlimited number of subsequent periods of 60 days each during the individual's lifetime and only, with respect to each such period, if the individual makes an election under this paragraph to receive hospice care under this part provided by, or under arrangements made by, a particular hospice program instead of certain other benefits under this title.

    (2)(A) Except as provided in subparagraphs (B) and (C) and except in such exceptional and unusual circumstances as the Secretary may provide, if an individual makes such an election for a period with respect to a particular hospice program, the individual shall be deemed to have waived all rights to have payment made under this title with respect to—

    (i) hospice care provided by another hospice program (other than under arrangements made by the particular hospice program) during the period, and

    (ii) services furnished during the period that are determined (in accordance with guidelines of the Secretary) to be—

        (I) related to the treatment of the individual's condition with respect to which a diagnosis of terminal illness has been made or

        (II) equivalent to (or duplicative of) hospice care;

            except that clause (ii) shall not apply to physicians' services furnished by the individual's attending physician (if not an employee of the hospice program) or to services provided by (or under arrangements made by) the hospice program.

(B) After an individual makes such an election with respect to a 90-day period or a subsequent 60-day period, the individual may revoke the election during the period, in which case—

    (i) the revocation shall act as a waiver of the right to have payment made under this part for any hospice care benefits for the remaining time in such period and (for purposes of subsection (a)(4) and subparagraph (A)) the individual shall be deemed to have been provided such benefits during such entire period, and

    (ii) the individual may at any time after the revocation execute a new election for a subsequent period, if the individual otherwise is entitled to hospice care benefits with respect to such a period.

(C) An individual may, once in each such period, change the hospice program with respect to which the election is made and such change shall not be considered a revocation of an election under subparagraph (B).

(D) For purposes of this title, an individual's election with respect to a hospice program shall no longer be considered to be in effect with respect to that hospice program after the date the individual's revocation or change of election with respect to that election takes effect.

(e) For purposes of subsections (b) and (c), inpatient hospital services, inpatient psychiatric hospital services, and post-hospital extended care services shall be taken into account only if payment is or would be, except for this section or the failure to comply with the request and certification requirements of or under section 1814(a), made with respect to such services under this part.

(f)(1) The Secretary shall provide for coverage, under clause (B) of subsection (a)(2), of extended care services which are not post-hospital extended care services at such time and for so long as the Secretary determines, and under such terms and conditions (described in paragraph (2)) as the Secretary finds appropriate, that the inclusion of such services will not result in any increase in the total of payments made under this title and will not alter the acute care nature of the benefit described in subsection (a)(2).

(2) The Secretary may provide—

   (A) for such limitations on the scope and extent of services described in subsection (a)(2)(B) and on the categories of individuals who may be eligible to receive such services, and

   (B) notwithstanding sections 1814, 1861(v), and 1886, for such restrictions and alternatives on the amounts and methods of payment for services described in such subsection,

      as may be necessary to carry out paragraph (1).

(g) For definition of "spell of illness," and for definitions of other terms used in this part, see section 1861.

Deductibles and Coinsurance

Sec. 1813. [42 U.S.C. 1395e]

(a)(1) The amount payable for inpatient hospital services or inpatient critical access hospital services furnished an individual during any spell of illness shall be reduced by a deduction equal to the inpatient hospital deductible or, if less, the charges imposed with respect to such individual for such services, except that, if the customary charges for such services are greater than the charges so imposed, such customary charges shall be considered to be the charges so imposed. Such amount shall be further reduced by a coinsurance amount equal to—

   (A) one-fourth of the inpatient hospital deductible for each day (before the 91st day) on which such individual is furnished such services during such spell of illness after such services have been furnished to him for 60 days during such spell; and

   (B) one-half of the inpatient hospital deductible for each day (before the day following the last day for which such individual is entitled under section 1812(a)(1) to have payment made on his behalf for inpatient hospital services or inpatient critical access hospital services during such spell of illness) on which such individual is furnished such services during such spell of illness after such services have been furnished to him for 90 days during such spell;

      except that the reduction under this sentence for any day shall not exceed the charges imposed for that day with respect to such individual for such services (and for this purpose, if the customary charges for such services are greater than the charges so imposed, such customary charges shall be considered to be the charges so imposed).

(2)(A) The amount payable to any provider of services under this part for services furnished an individual shall be further reduced by a deduction equal to the expenses incurred for the first three pints of whole blood (or equivalent quantities of packed red blood cells, as defined under regulations) furnished to the individual during each calendar year, except that such deductible for such blood shall in accordance with regulations be appropriately reduced to the extent that there has been a replacement of such blood (or equivalent quantities of packed red blood cells, as so defined); and for such purposes blood (or equivalent quantities of packed red blood cells, as so defined) furnished such individual shall be deemed replaced when the institution or other person furnishing such blood (or such equivalent quantities of packed red blood cells, as so defined) is given one pint of blood for each pint of blood (or equivalent quantities of packed red blood cells, as so defined) furnished such individual with respect to which a deduction is made under this sentence.

(B) The deductible under subparagraph (A) for blood or blood cells furnished an individual in a year shall be reduced to the extent that a deductible has been imposed under section 1833(b) to blood or blood cells furnished the individual in the year.

(3) The amount payable for post-hospital extended care services furnished an individual during any spell of illness shall be reduced by a coinsurance amount equal to one-eighth of the inpatient hospital deductible for each day (before the 101st day) on which he is furnished such services after such services have been furnished to him for 20 days during such spell.

(4)(A) The amount payable for hospice care shall be reduced—

(i) in the case of drugs and biologicals provided on an outpatient basis by (or under arrangements made by) the hospice program, by a coinsurance amount equal to an amount (not to exceed $5 per prescription) determined in accordance with a drug copayment schedule (established by the hospice program) which is related to, and approximates 5 percent of, the cost of the drug or biological to the program, and

(ii) in the case of respite care provided by (or under arrangements made by) the hospice program, by a coinsurance amount equal to 5 percent of the amount estimated by the hospice program (in accordance with regulations of the Secretary) to be equal to the amount of payment under section 1814(i) to that program for respite care; except that the total of the coinsurance required under clause (ii) for an individual may not exceed for a hospice coinsurance period the inpatient hospital deductible applicable for the year in which the period began. For purposes of this subparagraph, the term "hospice coinsurance period" means, for an individual, a period of consecutive days beginning with the first day for which an election under section 1812(d) is in effect for the individual and ending with the close of the first period of 14 consecutive days on each of which such an election is not in effect for the individual.

(B) During the period of an election by an individual under section 1812 (d)(1), no copayments or deductibles other than those under subparagraph (A) shall apply with respect to services furnished to such individual which constitute hospice care, regardless of the setting in which such services are furnished.

(b)(1) The inpatient hospital deductible for 1987 shall be $520. The inpatient hospital deductible for any succeeding year shall be an amount equal to the inpatient hospital deductible for the preceding calendar year, changed by the Secretary's best estimate of the payment-weighted average of the applicable percentage increases (as defined in section 1886(b)(3)(B)) which are applied under section 1886(d)(3)(A) for discharges in the fiscal year that begins on October 1 of such preceding calendar year, and adjusted to reflect changes in real case mix (determined on the basis of the most recent case mix data available). Any amount determined under the preceding sentence which is not a multiple of $4 shall be rounded to the nearest multiple of $4 (or, if it is midway between two multiples of $4, to the next higher multiple of $4).

(2) The Secretary shall promulgate the inpatient hospital deductible and all coinsurance amounts under this section between September 1 and September 15 of the year preceding the year to which they will apply.

(3) The inpatient hospital deductible for a year shall apply to—

   (A) the deduction under the first sentence of subsection (a)(1) for the year in which the first day of inpatient hospital services or inpatient critical access hospital services occurs in a spell of illness, and

   (B) to the coinsurance amounts under subsection (a) for inpatient hospital services, inpatient critical access hospital services and post-hospital extended care services furnished in that year.

Payment to Providers of Services

Sec. 1815. [42 U.S.C. 1395g]

(a) The Secretary shall periodically determine the amount which should be paid under this part to each provider of services with respect to the services furnished by it, and the provider of services shall be paid, at such time or times as the Secretary believes appropriate (but not less often than monthly) and prior to audit or settlement by the General Accounting Office,[18] from the Federal Hospital Insurance Trust Fund, the amounts so determined, with necessary adjustments on account of previously made overpayments or underpayments; except that no such payments shall be made to any provider unless it has furnished such information as the Secretary may request in order to determine the amounts due such provider under this part for the period with respect to which the amounts are being paid or any prior period.

(b) No payment shall be made to a provider of services which is a hospital for or with respect to services furnished by it for any period with respect to which it is deemed, under section 1861(w)(2), to have in effect an arrangement with a quality control and peer review organization for the conduct of utilization review activities by such organization unless such hospital has paid to such organization the amount due (as determined pursuant to such section) to such organization for the review activities conducted by it pursuant to such arrangements or such hospital has provided assurances satisfactory to the Secretary that such organization will promptly be paid the amount so due to it from the proceeds of the payment claimed by the hospital. Payment under this title for utilization review activities provided by a quality control and peer review organization pursuant to an arrangement or deemed arrangement with a hospital under section 1861(w)(2) shall be calculated without any requirement that the reasonable cost of such activities be apportioned among the patients of such hospital, if any, to whom such activities were not applicable.

(c) No payment which may be made to a provider of services under this title for any service furnished to an individual shall be made to any other person under an assignment or power of attorney; but nothing in this subsection shall be construed (1) to prevent the making of such a payment in accordance with an assignment from the provider if such assignment is made to a governmental agency or entity or is established by or pursuant to the order of a court of competent jurisdiction, or (2) to preclude an agent of the provider of services from receiving any such payment if (but only if) such agent does so pursuant to an agency agreement under which the compensation to be paid to the agent for his services for or in connection with the billing or collection of payments due such provider under this title is unrelated (directly or indirectly) to the amount of such payments or the billings therefor, and is not dependent upon the actual collection of any such payment.

(d) Whenever a final determination is made that the amount of payment made under this part to a provider of services was in excess of or less than the amount of payment that is due, and payment of such excess or deficit is not made (or effected by offset) within 30 days of the date of the determination, interest shall accrue on the balance of such excess or deficit not paid or offset (to the extent that the balance is owed by or owing to the provider) at a rate determined in accordance with the regulations of the Secretary of the Treasury applicable to charges for late payments.

(e)(1) The Secretary shall provide payment under this part for inpatient hospital services furnished by a subsection (d) hospital (as defined in section 1886(d)(1)(B), and including a distinct psychiatric or rehabilitation unit of such a hospital) and a subsection (d) Puerto Rico hospital (as defined in section 1886(d)(9)(A)) on a periodic interim payment basis (rather than on the basis of bills actually submitted) in the following cases:

(A) Upon the request of a hospital which is paid through an agency or organization with an agreement with the Secretary under section 1816, if the agency or organization, for three consecutive calendar months, fails to meet the requirements of subsection (c)(2) of such section and if the hospital meets the requirements (in effect as of October 1, 1986) applicable to payment on such a basis, until such time as the agency or organization meets such requirements for three consecutive calendar months.

(B) In the case of[19] hospital that—

(i) has a disproportionate share adjustment percentage (as established in clause (iv) of such section)[20] of at least 5.1 percent (as computed for purposes of establishing the average standardized amounts for discharges occurring during fiscal year 1987), and

(ii) requests payment on such basis,

but only if the hospital was being paid for inpatient hospital services on such a periodic interim payment basis as of June 30, 1987, and continues to meet the requirements (in effect as of October 1, 1986) applicable to payment on such a basis.

(C) In the case of a hospital that—

    (i) is located in a rural area,

    (ii) has 100 or fewer beds, and

    (iii) requests payment on such basis,

        but only if the hospital was being paid for inpatient hospital services on such a periodic interim payment basis as of June 30, 1987, and continues to meet the requirements (in effect as of October 1, 1986) applicable to payment on such a basis.

(2) The Secretary shall provide (or continue to provide) for payment on a periodic interim payment basis (under the standards established under section 405.454(j) of title 42, Code of Federal Regulations,[21] as in effect on October 1, 1986, in the cases described in subparagraphs (A) through (D)) with respect to—

(A) inpatient hospital services of a hospital that is not a subsection (d) hospital (as defined in section 1886(d)(1)(B));

(B) a hospital which is receiving payment under a State hospital reimbursement system under section 1814(b)(3) or 1886(c), if payment on a periodic interim payment basis is an integral part of such reimbursement system;

(C) extended care services;

(D) hospice care; and

(E)[22] inpatient critical access hospital services;

        if the provider of such services elects to receive, and qualifies for, such payments.

(3) In the case of a subsection (d) hospital or a subsection (d) Puerto Rico hospital (as defined for purposes of section 1886) which has significant cash flow problems resulting from operations of its intermediary or from unusual circumstances of the hospital's operation, the Secretary may make available appropriate accelerated payments.

(4) A hospital created by the merger or consolidation of 2 or more hospitals or hospital campuses shall be eligible to receive periodic interim payment on the basis described in paragraph (1)(B) if—

(A) at least one of the hospitals or campuses received periodic interim payment on such basis prior to the merger or consolidation; and

(B) the merging or consolidating hospitals or campuses would each meet the requirement of paragraph (1)(B)(i) if such hospitals or campuses were treated as independent hospitals for purposes of this title.

Provisions Relating to the Administration of Part A[23]

Sec. 1816. [42 U.S.C. 1395h]

(a) The administration of this part shall be conducted through contracts with medicare administrative contractors under section 1874A.

(b) [Repealed.[24]]

(c)(1) [Stricken.[25]]

    (2)(A) Each contract under section 1874A that provides for making payments under this part shall provide that payment shall be issued, mailed, or otherwise transmitted with respect to not less than 95 percent of all claims submitted under this title—

        (i) which are clean claims, and

        (ii) for which payment is not made on a periodic interim payment basis, within the applicable number of calendar days after the date on which the claim is received.

    (B) In this paragraph:

        (i) The term "clean claim" means a claim that has no defect or impropriety (including any lack of any required substantiating documentation) or particular circumstance requiring special treatment that prevents timely payment from being made on the claim under this title.

        (ii) The term "applicable number of calendar days" means—

            (I) with respect to claims received in the 12-month period beginning October 1, 1986, 30 calendar days,

            (II) with respect to claims received in the 12-month period beginning October 1, 1987, 26 calendar days,

            (III) with respect to claims received in the 12-month period beginning October 1, 1988, 25 calendar days,

            (IV) with respect to claims received in the 12-month period beginning October 1, 1989, and claims received in any succeeding 12-month period ending on or before September 30, 1993, 24 calendar days, and

            (V) with respect to claims received in the 12-month period beginning October 1, 1993, and claims received in any succeeding 12-month period, 30 calendar days.

    (C) If payment is not issued, mailed, or otherwise transmitted within the applicable number of calendar days (as defined in clause (ii) of subparagraph (B)) after a clean claim (as defined in clause (i) of such subparagraph) is received from a hospital, critical access hospital, skilled nursing facility, home health agency, hospice program, comprehensive outpatient rehabilitation facility, or rehabilitation agency that is not receiving payments on a periodic interim payment basis with respect to such services, interest shall be paid at the rate used for purposes of section 3902(a) of title 31, United States Code[26] (relating to interest penalties for failure to make prompt payments) for the period beginning on the day after the required payment date and ending on the date on which payment is made.

    (3)(A) Each contract under section 1874A that provides for making payments under this part shall provide that no payment shall be issued, mailed, or otherwise transmitted with respect to any claim submitted under this title within the applicable number of calendar days after the date on which the claim is received.

(B) In this paragraph, the term "applicable number of calendar days" means—
    (i) with respect to claims submitted electronically as prescribed by the Secretary, 13 days, and
    (ii) with respect to claims submitted otherwise, 28 days.

(d)(i) [Repealed.[27]]

(j) A contract with a medicare administrative contractor under section 1874A with respect to the administration of this part shall require that, with respect to a claim for home health services, extended care services, or post-hospital extended care services submitted by a provider to such agency or organization that is denied, such agency or organization—
    (1) furnish the provider and the individual with respect to whom the claim is made with a written explanation of the denial and of the statutory or regulatory basis for the denial; and
    (2) in the case of a request for reconsideration of a denial, promptly notify such individual and the provider of the disposition of such reconsideration.

(k) A contract with a medicare administrative contractor under section 1874A with respect to the administration of this part shall require that such medicare administrative contractor submit an annual report to the Secretary describing the steps taken to recover payments made for items or services for which payment has been or could be made under a primary plan (as defined in section 1862(b)(2)(A)).

Federal Hospital Insurance Trust Fund[28]

Sec. 1817. [42 U.S.C. 1395i]

(a) There is hereby created on the books of the Treasury of the United States a trust fund to be known as the "Federal Hospital Insurance Trust Fund" (hereinafter in this section referred to as the "Trust Fund"). The Trust Fund shall consist of such gifts and bequests as may be made as provided in section 201(i)(1), and such amounts as may be deposited in, or appropriated to, such fund as provided in this part. There are hereby appropriated to the Trust Fund for the fiscal year ending June 30, 1966, and for each fiscal year thereafter, out of any moneys in the Treasury not otherwise appropriated, amounts equivalent to 100 per centum of—
(1) the taxes imposed by sections 3101(b) and 3111(b) of the Internal Revenue Code of 1954[29] with respect to wages reported to the Secretary of the Treasury or his delegate pursuant to subtitle F of such Code[30] after December 31, 1965, as determined by the Secretary of the Treasury by applying the applicable rates of tax under such sections to such wages, which wages shall be certified by the Commissioner of Social Security on the basis of records of wages established and maintained by the Commissioner of Social Security in accordance with such reports; and
(2) the taxes imposed by section 1401(b) of the Internal Revenue Code of 1954[31] with respect to self-employment income reported to the Secretary of the Treasury or his delegate on tax returns under subtitle F of such Code, as determined by the Secretary of the Treasury by applying

the applicable rate of tax under such section to such self-employment income, which self-employment income shall be certified by the Commissioner of Social Security on the basis of records of self-employment established and maintained by the Commissioner of Social Security in accordance with such returns.

The amounts appropriated by the preceding sentence shall be transferred from time to time from the general fund in the Treasury to the Trust Fund, such amounts to be determined on the basis of estimates by the Secretary of the Treasury of the taxes, specified in the preceding sentence, paid to or deposited into the Treasury; and proper adjustments shall be made in amounts subsequently transferred to the extent prior estimates were in excess of or were less than the taxes specified in such sentence.

(b) With respect to the Trust Fund, there is hereby created a body to be known as the Board of Trustees of the Trust Fund (hereinafter in this section referred to as the "Board of Trustees") composed of the Commissioner of Social Security, the Secretary of the Treasury, the Secretary of Labor, and the Secretary of Health and Human Services, all ex officio, and of two members of the public (both of whom may not be from the same political party), who shall be nominated by the President for a term of four years and subject to confirmation by the Senate. A member of the Board of Trustees serving as a member of the public and nominated and confirmed to fill a vacancy occurring during a term shall be nominated and confirmed only for the remainder of such term. An individual nominated and confirmed as a member of the public may serve in such position after the expiration of such member's term until the earlier of the time at which the member's successor takes office or the time at which a report of the Board is first issued under paragraph (2) after the expiration of the member's term. The Secretary of the Treasury shall be the Managing Trustee of the Board of Trustees (hereinafter in this section referred to as the "Managing Trustee"). The Administrator of the Centers for Medicare and Medicaid Services shall serve as the Secretary of the Board of Trustees. The Board of Trustees shall meet not less frequently than once each calendar year. It shall be the duty of the Board of Trustees to—

(1) Hold the Trust Fund;

(2) Report to the Congress not later than the first day of April of each year on the operation and status of the Trust Fund during the preceding fiscal year and on its expected operation and status during the current fiscal year and the next 2 fiscal years;

Each report provided under paragraph (2) beginning with the report in 2005 shall include the information specified in section 801(a) of the Medicare Prescription Drug, Improvement, and Modernization Act of 2003.[32]

(3) Report immediately to the Congress whenever the Board is of the opinion that the amount of the Trust Fund is unduly small; and

(4) Review the general policies followed in managing the Trust Fund, and recommend changes in such policies, including necessary changes in

the provisions of law which govern the way in which the Trust Fund is to be managed.

The report provided for in paragraph (2) shall include a statement of the assets of, and the disbursements made from, the Trust Fund during the preceding fiscal year, an estimate of the expected income to, and disbursements to be made from, the Trust Fund during the current fiscal year and each of the next 2 fiscal years, and a statement of the actuarial status of the Trust Fund. Such report shall also include an actuarial opinion by the Chief Actuary of the Centers for Medicare and Medicaid Services certifying that the techniques and methodologies used are generally accepted within the actuarial profession and that the assumptions and cost estimates used are reasonable. Such report shall be printed as a House document of the session of the Congress to which the report is made. A person serving on the Board of Trustees shall not be considered to be a fiduciary and shall not be personally liable for actions taken in such capacity with respect to the Trust Fund.

(c) It shall be the duty of the Managing Trustee to invest such portion of the Trust Fund as is not, in his judgment, required to meet current withdrawals. Such investments may be made only in interest-bearing obligations of the United States or in obligations guaranteed as to both principal and interest by the United States. For such purpose such obligations may be acquired (1) on original issue at the issue price, or (2) by purchase of outstanding obligations at the market price. The purposes for which obligations of the United States may be issued under chapter 31 of title 31, United States Code,[33] are hereby extended to authorize the issuance at par of public-debt obligations for purchase by the Trust Fund. Such obligations issued for purchase by the Trust Fund shall have maturities fixed with due regard for the needs of the Trust Fund and shall bear interest at a rate equal to the average market yield (computed by the Managing Trustee on the basis of market quotations as of the end of the calendar month next preceding the date of such issue) on all marketable interest-bearing obligations of the United States then forming a part of the public debt which are not due or callable until after the expiration of 4 years from the end of such calendar month; except that where such average market yield is not a multiple of one-eighth of 1 per centum, the rate of interest on such obligations shall be the multiple of one-eighth of 1 per centum nearest such market yield. The Managing Trustee may purchase other interest-bearing obligations of the United States or obligations guaranteed as to both principal and interest by the United States, on original issue or at the market price, only where he determines that the purchase of such other obligations is in the public interest.

(d) Any obligations acquired by the Trust Fund (except public-debt obligations issued exclusively to the Trust Fund) may be sold by the Managing Trustee at the market price, and such public-debt obligations may be redeemed at par plus accrued interest.

(e) The interest on, and the proceeds from the sale or redemption of, any obligations held in the Trust Fund shall be credited to and form a part of the Trust Fund.

(f)(1) The Managing Trustee is directed to pay from time to time from the Trust Fund into the Treasury the amount estimated by him as taxes imposed under section 3101(b) which are subject to refund under section 6413(c) of the Internal Revenue Code of 1954[34] with respect to wages paid after December 31, 1965. Such taxes shall be determined on the basis of the records of wages established and maintained by the Commissioner of Social Security in accordance with the wages reported to the Secretary of the Treasury or his delegate pursuant to subtitle F of the Internal Revenue Code of 1954,[35] and the Commissioner of Social Security shall furnish the Managing Trustee such information as may be required by the Managing Trustee for such purpose. The payments by the Managing Trustee shall be covered into the Treasury as repayments to the account for refunding internal revenue collections.

(2) Repayments made under paragraph (1) shall not be available for expenditures but shall be carried to the surplus fund of the Treasury. If it subsequently appears that the estimates under such paragraph in any particular period were too high or too low, appropriate adjustments shall be made by the Managing Trustee in future payments.

(g) There shall be transferred periodically (but not less often than once each fiscal year) to the Trust Fund from the Federal Old-Age and Survivors Insurance Trust Fund and from the Federal Disability Insurance Trust Fund amounts equivalent to the amounts not previously so transferred which the Secretary of Health and Human Services shall have certified as overpayments (other than amounts so certified to the Railroad Retirement Board) pursuant to section 1870(b) of this Act. There shall be transferred periodically (but not less often than once each fiscal year) to the Trust Fund from the Railroad Retirement Account amounts equivalent to the amounts not previously so transferred which the Secretary of Health and Human Services shall have certified as overpayments to the Railroad Retirement Board pursuant to section 1870(b) of this Act.

(h) The Managing Trustee shall also pay from time to time from the Trust Fund such amounts as the Secretary of Health and Human Services certifies are necessary to make the payments provided for by this part, and the payments with respect to administrative expenses in accordance with section 201(g)(1).

(i) There are authorized to be made available for expenditure out of the Trust Fund such amounts as are required to pay travel expenses, either on an actual cost or commuted basis, to parties, their representatives, and all reasonably necessary witnesses for travel within the United States (as defined in section 210(i)) to attend reconsideration interviews and proceedings before administrative law judges with respect to any determination under this title. The amount available under the preceding sentence for payment for air travel by any person shall not exceed the coach fare for air travel between the points involved unless the use of first-class accommodations is required (as determined under regulations of the Secretary) because of such person's health condition or the unavailability of alternative accommodations; and the amount available for payment for other travel by any person shall not exceed the cost of travel (between the points involved) by the most economical and expeditious means of transportation appropriate to such person's health condition, as specified in such regulations. The amount available for payment under this subsection for travel by a representative to attend an administrative proceeding before an administrative law judge or other adjudicator shall not exceed the maximum amount allowable under this subsection for such travel originating within the geographic area of the office having jurisdiction over such proceeding.

(j)(1) If at any time prior to January 1988 the Managing Trustee determines that borrowing authorized under this subsection is appropriate in order to best meet the need for financing the benefit payments from the Federal Hospital Insurance Trust Fund, the Managing Trustee may, subject to paragraph (5), borrow such amounts as he determines to be appropriate from either the Federal Old-Age and Survivors Insurance Trust Fund or the Federal Disability Insurance Trust Fund for transfer to and deposit in the Federal Hospital Insurance Trust Fund.

(2) In any case where a loan has been made to the Federal Hospital Insurance Trust Fund under paragraph (1), there shall be transferred on the last day of each month after such loan is made, from such Trust Fund to the lending Trust Fund, the total interest accrued to such day with respect to the unrepaid balance of such loan at a rate equal to the rate which the lending Trust Fund would earn on the amount involved if the loan were an investment under subsection (c) (even if such an investment would earn interest at a rate different than the rate earned by investments redeemed by the lending fund in order to make the loan).

(3)(A) If in any month after a loan has been made to the Federal Hospital Insurance Trust Fund under paragraph (1), the Managing Trustee determines that the assets of such Trust Fund are sufficient to permit repayment of all or part of any loans made to such Fund under paragraph (1), he shall make such repayments as he determines to be appropriate.

(B)(i) If on the last day of any year after a loan has been made under paragraph (1) by the Federal Old-Age and Survivors Insurance Trust Fund or the Federal Disability Insurance Trust Fund to the Federal Hospital Insurance Trust Fund, the Managing Trustee determines that the Hospital Insurance Trust Fund ratio exceeds 15 percent, he shall transfer from such Trust Fund to the lending trust fund an amount that—

(I) together with any amounts transferred to another lending trust fund under this paragraph for such year, will reduce the Hospital Insurance Trust Fund ratio to 15 percent; and

(II) does not exceed the outstanding balance of such loan.

(ii) Amounts required to be transferred under clause (i) shall be transferred on the last day of the first month of the year succeeding the year in which the determination described in clause (i) is made.

(iii) For purposes of this subparagraph, the term "Hospital Insurance Trust Fund ratio" means, with respect to any calendar year, the ratio of—

   (I) the balance in the Federal Hospital Insurance Trust Fund, as of the last day of such calendar year; to

   (II) the amount estimated by the Secretary to be the total amount to be paid from the Federal Hospital Insurance Trust Fund during the calendar year following such calendar year (other than payments of interest on, and repayments of, loans from the Federal Old-Age and Survivors Insurance Trust Fund and the Federal Disability Insurance Trust Fund under paragraph (1)), and reducing the amount of any transfer to the Railroad Retirement Account by the amount of any transfers into such Trust Fund from the Railroad Retirement Account.

(C)(i) The full amount of all loans made under paragraph (1) (whether made before or after January 1, 1983) shall be repaid at the earliest feasible date and in any event no later than December 31, 1989.

   (ii) For the period after December 31, 1987 and before January 1, 1990, the Managing Trustee shall transfer each month from the Federal Hospital Insurance Trust Fund to any Trust Fund that is owed any amount by the Federal Hospital Insurance Trust Fund on a loan made under paragraph (1), an amount not less than an amount equal to (I) the amount owed to such Trust Fund by the Federal Hospital Insurance Trust Fund at the beginning of such month (plus the interest accrued on the outstanding balance of such loan during such month), divided by (II) the number of months elapsing after the preceding month and before January 1990. The Managing Trustee may, during this period, transfer larger amounts than prescribed by the preceding sentence.

(4) The Board of Trustees shall make a timely report to the Congress of any amounts transferred (including interest payments) under this subsection.

(5)(A) No amounts may be loaned by the Federal Old-Age and Survivors Insurance Trust Fund or the Federal Disability Insurance Trust Fund under paragraph (1) during any month if the OASDI trust fund ratio for such month is less than 10 percent.

(B) For purposes of this paragraph, the term "OASDI trust fund ratio" means, with respect to any month, the ratio of—

   (i) the combined balance in the Federal Old-Age and Survivors Insurance Trust Fund and the Federal Disability Insurance Trust Fund, reduced by the outstanding amount of any loan (including interest thereon) theretofore made to either such Trust Fund from the Federal Hospital Insurance Trust Fund under section 201(l), as of the last day of the second month preceding such month, to

   (ii) the amount obtained by multiplying by twelve the total amount which (as estimated by the Secretary) will be paid from the Federal Old-Age and Survivors Insurance Trust Fund and the Federal Disability Insurance Trust Fund during the month for which such ratio is to be determined for all purposes authorized by section 201 (other than payments of interest on, or repayments of, loans from the Federal Hospital Insurance Trust Fund under section 201(l)), but excluding any transfer payments between such trust funds and reducing the amount of any transfers to the Railroad Retirement Account by the amount of any transfers into either such trust fund from that Account.

(k) Health Care Fraud and Abuse Control Account.—

    (1) Establishment.—There is hereby established in the Trust Fund an expenditure account to be known as the "Health Care Fraud and Abuse Control Account" (in this subsection referred to as the "Account").

    (2) Appropriated amounts to trust fund.—

        (A) In general.—There are hereby appropriated to the Trust Fund—

            (i) such gifts and bequests as may be made as provided in subparagraph (B);

            (ii) such amounts as may be deposited in the Trust Fund as provided in sections 242(b) and 249(c) of the Health Insurance Portability and Accountability Act of 1996[36], and title XI; and

            (iii) such amounts as are transferred to the Trust Fund under subparagraph (C).

        (B) Authorization to accept gifts.—The Trust Fund is authorized to accept on behalf of the United States money gifts and bequests made unconditionally to the Trust Fund, for the benefit of the Account or any activity financed through the Account.

        (C) Transfer of amounts.—The Managing Trustee shall transfer to the Trust Fund, under rules similar to the rules in section 9601 of the Internal Revenue Code of 1986,[37] an amount equal to the sum of the following:

            (i) Criminal fines recovered in cases involving a Federal health care offense (as defined in section 24(a) of title 18, United States Code[38]).

            (ii) Civil monetary penalties and assessments imposed in health care cases, including amounts recovered under titles XI, XVIII, and XIX, and chapter 38 of title 31, United States Code (except as otherwise provided by law).

            (iii) Amounts resulting from the forfeiture of property by reason of a Federal health care offense.

            (iv) Penalties and damages obtained and otherwise creditable to miscellaneous receipts of the general fund of the Treasury obtained under sections 3729 through 3733 of title 31, United States Code (known as the False Claims Act), in cases involving claims related to the provision of health care items and services (other than funds awarded to a relator, for restitution or otherwise authorized by law).

        (D) Application.—Nothing in subparagraph (C)(iii) shall be construed to limit the availability of recoveries and forfeitures obtained under title I of the Employee Retirement Income Security Act of 1974 for the purpose of providing equitable or remedial relief for employee welfare benefit plans, and for participants and beneficiaries under such plans, as authorized under such title.

(3) Appropriated amounts to account for fraud and abuse control program, etc.—

(A) Departments of health and human services and justice.—

(i) In general.—There are hereby appropriated to the Account from the Trust Fund such sums as the Secretary and the Attorney General certify are necessary to carry out the purposes described in subparagraph (C), to be available without further appropriation until expended, in an amount not to exceed—

(I) for fiscal year 1997, $104,000,000.

(II) for each of the fiscal years 1998 through 2003, the limit for the preceding fiscal year, increased by 15 percent;

(III) for each of fiscal years 2004, 2005, and 2006, the limit for fiscal year 2003;

(IV) for each of fiscal years 2007, 2008, 2009, and 2010, the limit under this clause for the preceding fiscal year, increased by the percentage increase in the consumer price index for all urban consumers (all items; United States city average) over the previous year; and

(V) for each fiscal year after fiscal year 2010, the limit under this clause for fiscal year 2010.

(ii) Medicare and medicaid activities.—For each fiscal year, of the amount appropriated in clause (i), the following amounts shall be available only for the purposes of the activities of the Office of the Inspector General of the Department of Health and Human Services with respect to the Medicare and medicaid programs—

(I) for fiscal year 1997, not less than $60,000,000 and not more than $70,000,000;

(II) for fiscal year 1998, not less than $80,000,000 and not more than $90,000,000;

(III) for fiscal year 1999, not less than $90,000,000 and not more than $100,000,000;

(IV) for fiscal year 2000, not less than $110,000,000 and not more than $120,000,000;

(V) for fiscal year 2001, not less than $120,000,000 and not more than $130,000,000;

(VI) for fiscal year 2002, not less than $140,000,000 and not more than $150,000,000;

(VII) for each of fiscal years 2003, 2004, 2005, and 2006, not less than $150,000,000 and not more than $160,000,000;

(VIII) for fiscal year 2007, not less than $160,000,000, increased by the percentage increase in the consumer price index for all urban consumers (all items; United States city average) over the previous year;

(IX) for each of fiscal years 2008, 2009, and 2010, not less than the amount required under this clause for the preceding fiscal year, increased by the percentage increase in the consumer price index for all urban consumers (all items; United States city average) over the previous year; and

(X) for each fiscal year after fiscal year 2010, not less than the amount required under this clause for fiscal year 2010.

(B) Federal Bureau of Investigation.—There are hereby appropriated from the general fund of the United States Treasury and hereby appropriated to the Account for transfer to the Federal Bureau of Investigation to carry out the purposes described in subparagraph (C), to be available without further appropriation until expended—

(i) for fiscal year 1997, $47,000,000;

(ii) for fiscal year 1998, $56,000,000;

(iii) for fiscal year 1999, $66,000,000;

(iv) for fiscal year 2000, $76,000,000;

(v) for fiscal year 2001, $88,000,000;

(vi) for fiscal year 2002, $101,000,000;

(vii) for each of fiscal years 2003, 2004, 2005, and 2006, $114,000,000;

(viii) for each of fiscal years 2007, 2008, 2009, and 2010, the amount to be appropriated under this subparagraph for the preceding fiscal year, increased by the percentage increase in the consumer price index for all urban consumers (all items; United States city average) over the previous year; and

(ix) for each fiscal year after fiscal year 2010, the amount to be appropriated under this subparagraph for fiscal year 2010.

(C) Use of funds.—The purposes described in this subparagraph are to cover the costs (including equipment, salaries and benefits, and travel and training) of the administration and operation of the health care fraud and abuse control program established under section 1128C (a), including the costs of—

(i) prosecuting health care matters (through criminal, civil, and administrative proceedings);

(ii) investigations;

(iii) financial and performance audits of health care programs and operations;

(iv) inspections and other evaluations; and

(v) provider and consumer education regarding compliance with the provisions of title XI.

(4) Appropriated amounts to account for Medicare integrity program.—

(A) In general.—There are hereby appropriated to the Account from the Trust Fund for each fiscal year such amounts as are necessary to carry out the Medicare Integrity Program under section 1893, subject to subparagraph (B), (C) and (D) and to be available without further appropriation.

(B) Amounts specified.—Subject to subparagraph (C), the amount appropriated under subparagraph (A) for a fiscal year is as follows:

(i) For fiscal year 1997, such amount shall be not less than $430,000,000 and not more than $440,000,000.

(ii) For fiscal year 1998, such amount shall be not less than $490,000,000 and not more than $500,000,000.

(iii) For fiscal year 1999, such amount shall be not less than $550,000,000 and not more than $560,000,000.

(iv) For fiscal year 2000, such amount shall be not less than $620,000,000 and not more than $630,000,000.

(v) For fiscal year 2001, such amount shall be not less than $670,000,000 and not more than $680,000,000.

(vi) For fiscal year 2002, such amount shall be not less than $690,000,000 and not more than $700,000,000.

(vii) For each fiscal year after fiscal year 2002, such amount shall be not less than $710,000,000 and not more than $720,000,000.

(C) Adjustments.—The amount appropriated under subparagraph (A) for a fiscal year is increased as follows:

(i) For fiscal year 2006, $100,000,000.

(D) Expansion of the medicare-medicaid data match program.—The amount appropriated under subparagraph (A) for a fiscal year is further increased as follows for purposes of carrying out section 1893 (b)(6) for the respective fiscal year:

(i) $12,000,000 for fiscal year 2006.

(ii) $24,000,000 for fiscal year 2007.

(5) Annual report.—Not later than January 1, the Secretary and the Attorney General shall submit jointly a report to Congress which identifies—

(A) the amounts appropriated to the Trust Fund for the previous fiscal year under paragraph (2)(A) and the source of such amounts; and

(B) the amounts appropriated from the Trust Fund for such year under paragraph (3) and the justification for the expenditure of such amounts.

(6) GAO report.—Not later than June 1, 1998, and January 1 of 2000, 2002, and 2004, the Comptroller General of the United States shall submit a report to Congress which—

(A) identifies—

(i) the amounts appropriated to the Trust Fund for the previous two fiscal years under paragraph (2)(A) and the source of such amounts; and

(ii) the amounts appropriated from the Trust Fund for such fiscal years under paragraph (3) and the justification for the expenditure of such amounts;

(B) identifies any expenditures from the Trust Fund with respect to activities not involving the program under this title;

(C) identifies any savings to the Trust Fund, and any other savings, resulting from expenditures from the Trust Fund; and

(D) analyzes such other aspects of the operation of the Trust Fund as the Comptroller General of the United States considers appropriate.

Hospital Insurance Benefits for Uninsured Elderly Individuals Not Otherwise Eligible

Sec. 1818. [42 U.S.C. 1395i–2]

(a) Every individual who—
(1) has attained the age of 65,
(2) is enrolled under part B of this title,
(3) is a resident of the United States, and is either (A) a citizen or (B) an alien lawfully admitted for permanent residence who has resided in the United States continuously during the 5 years immediately preceding the month in which he applies for enrollment under this section, and
(4) is not otherwise entitled to benefits under this part,
shall be eligible to enroll in the insurance program established by this part. Except as otherwise provided, any reference to an individual entitled to benefits under this part includes an individual entitled to benefits under this part pursuant to an enrollment under this section or section 1818A.
(b) An individual may enroll under this section only in such manner and form as may be prescribed in regulations, and only during an enrollment period prescribed in or under this section.
(c) The provisions of section 1837 (except subsection (f) thereof), section 1838, subsection (b) of section 1839, and subsections (f) and (h) of section 1840 shall apply to persons authorized to enroll under this section except that—
(1) individuals who meet the conditions of subsection (a)(1), (3), and (4) on or before the last day of the seventh month after the month in which this section is enacted[39] may enroll under this part and (if not already so enrolled) may also enroll under part B during an initial general enrollment period which shall begin on the first day of the second month which begins after the date on which this section is enacted and shall end on the last day of the tenth month after the month in which this section is enacted;
(2) in the case of an individual who first meets the conditions of eligibility under this section on or after the first day of the eighth month after the month in which this section is enacted, the initial enrollment period shall begin on the first day of the third month before the month in which he first becomes eligible and shall end 7 months later;
(3) in the case of an individual who enrolls pursuant to paragraph (1) of this subsection, entitlement to benefits shall begin on—
(A) the first day of the second month after the month in which he enrolls,
(B) July 1, 1973, or
(C) the first day of the first month in which he meets the requirements of subsection (a),
whichever is the latest;
(4) an individual's entitlement under this section shall terminate with the month before the first month in which he becomes eligible for hospital insurance benefits under section 226 of this Act or section 103 of the Social Security Amendments of 1965[40]; and upon such termination, such individual shall be deemed, solely for purposes of hospital

insurance entitlement, to have filed in such first month the application required to establish such entitlement;

(5) termination of coverage for supplementary medical insurance shall result in simultaneous termination of hospital insurance benefits for uninsured individuals who are not otherwise entitled to benefits under this Act;

(6) any percent increase effected under section 1839(b) in an individual's monthly premium may not exceed 10 percent and shall only apply to premiums paid during a period equal to twice the number of months in the full 12-month periods described in that section and shall be subject to reduction in accordance with subsection (d)(6);

(7) an individual who meets the conditions of subsection (a) may enroll under this part during a special enrollment period that includes any month during any part of which the individual is enrolled under section 1876 with an eligible organization and ending with the last day of the 8th consecutive month in which the individual is at no time so enrolled;

(8) in the case of an individual who enrolls during a special enrollment period under paragraph (7)—

(A) in any month of the special enrollment period in which the individual is at any time enrolled under section 1876 with an eligible organization or in the first month following such a month, the coverage period shall begin on the first day of the month in which the individual so enrolls (or, at the option of the individual, on the first day of any of the following three months), or

(B) in any other month of the special enrollment period, the coverage period shall begin on the first day of the month following the month in which the individual so enrolls; and

(9) in applying the provisions of section 1839(b), there shall not be taken into account months for which the individual can demonstrate that the individual was enrolled under section 1876 with an eligible organization.

(d)(1) The Secretary shall, during September of each year (beginning with 1988), estimate the monthly actuarial rate for months in the succeeding year. Such actuarial rate shall be one-twelfth of the amount which the Secretary estimates (on an average, per capita basis) is equal to 100 percent of the benefits and administrative costs which will be payable from the Federal Hospital Insurance Trust Fund for services performed and related administrative costs incurred in the succeeding year with respect to individuals age 65 and over who will be entitled to benefits under this part during that year.

(2) The Secretary shall, during September of each year determine and promulgate the dollar amount which shall be applicable for premiums for months occurring in the following year. Subject to paragraphs (4) and (5), the amount of an individual's monthly premium under this section shall be equal to the monthly actuarial rate determined under paragraph (1) for that following year. Any amount determined under the preceding sentence which is not a multiple of $1 shall be rounded to

the nearest multiple of $1 (or, if it is a multiple of 50 cents but not a multiple of $1, to the next higher multiple of $1).

(3) Whenever the Secretary promulgates the dollar amount which shall be applicable as the monthly premium under this section, he shall, at the time such promulgation is announced, issue a public statement setting forth the actuarial assumptions and bases employed by him in arriving at the amount of an adequate actuarial rate for individuals 65 and older as provided in paragraph (1).

(4)(A) In the case of an individual described in subparagraph (B), the monthly premium for a month shall be reduced by the applicable reduction percent specified in the following table:

For a month in:	The applicable reduction percent is:
1994	25 percent
1995	30 percent
1996	35 percent
1997	40 percent
1998 or subsequent year	45 percent.

(B) An individual described in this subparagraph with respect to a month is an individual who establishes to the satisfaction of the Secretary that, as of the last day of the previous month, the individual—

(i) had at least 30 quarters of coverage under title II;

(ii) was married (and had been married for the previous 1-year period) to an individual who had at least 30 quarters of coverage under such title;

(iii) had been married to an individual for a period of at least 1 year (at the time of such individual's death) if at such time the individual had at least 30 quarters of coverage under such title; or

(iv) is divorced from an individual and had been married to the individual for a period of at least 10 years (at the time of the divorce) if at such time the individual had at least 30 quarters of coverage under such title.

(5)(A) The amount of the monthly premium shall be zero in the case of an individual who is a person described in subparagraph (B) for a month, if—

(i) the individual's premium under this section for the month is not (and will not be) paid for, in whole or in part, by a State (under title XIX or otherwise), a political subdivision of a State, or an agency or instrumentality of one or more States or political subdivisions thereof; and

(ii) in each of 84 months before such month, the individual was enrolled in this part under this section and the payment of the individual's premium under this section for the month was not paid for, in whole or in part, by a State (under title XIX or otherwise), a political subdivision of a State, or an agency or instrumentality of one or more States or political subdivisions thereof.

(B) A person described in this subparagraph for a month is a person who establishes to the satisfaction of the Secretary that, as of the last day of the previous month—

(i)(I) the person was receiving cash benefits under a qualified State or local government retirement system (as defined in subparagraph (C)) on the basis of the person's employment in one or more positions covered under any such system, and (II) the person would have at least 40 quarters of coverage under title II if remuneration for medicare qualified government employment (as defined in paragraph (1) of section 210(p), but determined without regard to paragraph (3) of such section) paid to such person were treated as wages paid to such person and credited for purposes of determining quarters of coverage under section 213;

(ii)(I) the person was married (and had been married for the previous 1-year period) to an individual who is described in clause (i), or (II) the person met the requirement of clause (i)(II) and was married (and had been married for the previous 1-year period) to an individual described in clause (i)(I);

(iii) the person had been married to an individual for a period of at least 1 year (at the time of such individual's death) if (I) the individual was described in clause (i) at the time of the individual's death, or (II) the person met the requirement of clause (i)(II) and the individual was described in clause (i)(I) at the time of the individual's death; or

(iv) the person is divorced from an individual and had been married to the individual for a period of at least 10 years (at the time of the divorce) if (I) the individual was described in clause (i) at the time of the divorce, or (II) the person met the requirement of clause (i)(II) and the individual was described in clause (i)(I) at the time of the divorce.

(C) For purposes of subparagraph (B)(i)(I), the term "qualified State or local government retirement system" means a retirement system that—

(i) is established or maintained by a State or political subdivision thereof, or an agency or instrumentality of one or more States or political subdivisions thereof;

(ii) covers positions of some or all employees of such a State, subdivision, agency, or instrumentality; and

(iii) does not adjust cash retirement benefits based on eligibility for a reduction in premium under this paragraph.

(6)(A) In the case where a State, a political subdivision of a State, or an agency or instrumentality of a State or political subdivision thereof determines to pay, for the life of each individual, the monthly premiums due under paragraph (1) on behalf of each of the individuals in a qualified State or local government retiree group who meets the conditions of subsection (a), the amount of any increase otherwise applicable under section 1839(b) (as applied and modified by subsection (c)(6) of this section) with respect to the monthly premium for benefits under this part for an individual who is a member of such group shall be reduced by the total amount of taxes paid under section 3101(b) of the Internal Revenue Code of 1986 by such individual and under 3111(b) of such Code by the employers of such individual on behalf of such individual with respect to employment (as defined in section 3121(b) of such Code).

(B) For purposes of this paragraph, the term "qualified State or local government retiree group" means all of the individuals who retire prior to a specified date that is before January 1, 2002, from employment in one or more occupations or other broad classes of employees of—
(i) the State;
(ii) a political subdivision of the State; or
(iii) an agency or instrumentality of the State or political subdivision of the State.

(e) Payment of the monthly premiums on behalf of any individual who meets the conditions of subsection (a) may be made by any public or private agency or organization under a contract or other arrangement entered into between it and the Secretary if the Secretary determines that payment of such premiums under such contract or arrangement is administratively feasible.

(f) Amounts paid to the Secretary for coverage under this section shall be deposited in the Treasury to the credit of the Federal Hospital Insurance Trust Fund.

(g)(1) The Secretary shall, at the request of a State made after 1989, enter into a modification of an agreement entered into with the State pursuant to section 1843(a) under which the agreement provides for enrollment in the program established by this part of qualified medicare beneficiaries (as defined in section 1905(p)(1)).

(2)(A) Except as provided in subparagraph (B), the provisions of subsections (c), (d), (e), and (f) of section 1843 shall apply to qualified medicare beneficiaries enrolled, pursuant to such agreement, in the program established by this part in the same manner and to the same extent as they apply to qualified medicare beneficiaries enrolled, pursuant to such agreement, in part B.

(B) For purposes of this subsection, section 1843(d)(1) shall be applied by substituting "section 1818" for "section 1839" and "subsection (c)(6) (with reference to subsection (b) of section 1839)" for "subsection (b)."

Hospital Insurance Benefits for Disabled Individuals Who Have Exhausted Other Entitlement

Sec. 1818A. [42 U.S.C. 1395i–2a]

(a) Every individual who—
(1) has not attained the age of 65;
(2)(A) has been entitled to benefits under this part under section 226(b), and

(B)(i) continues to have the disabling physical or mental impairment on the basis of which the individual was found to be under a disability or to be a disabled qualified railroad retirement beneficiary, or (ii) is blind (within the meaning of section 216(i)(1)), but

(C) whose entitlement under section 226(b) ends due solely to the individual having earnings that exceed the substantial gainful activity amount (as defined in section 223(d)(4)); and

(3) is not otherwise entitled to benefits under this part,

shall be eligible to enroll in the insurance program established by this part.

(b)(1) An individual may enroll under this section only in such manner and form as may be prescribed in regulations, and only during an enrollment period prescribed in or under this section.

(2) The individual's initial enrollment period shall begin with the month in which the individual receives notice that the individual's entitlement to benefits under section 226(b) will end due solely to the individual having earnings that exceed the substantial gainful activity amount (as defined in section 223(d)(4)) and shall end 7 months later.

(3) There shall be a general enrollment period during the period beginning on January 1 and ending on March 31 of each year (beginning with 1990).

(c)(1) The period (in this subsection referred to as a "coverage period") during which an individual is entitled to benefits under the insurance program under this part shall begin on whichever of the following is the latest:

(A) In the case of an individual who enrolls under subsection (b)(2) before the month in which the individual first satisfies subsection (a), the first day of such month.

(B) In the case of an individual who enrolls under subsection (b)(2) in the month in which the individual first satisfies subsection (a), the first day of the month following the month in which the individual so enrolls.

(C) In the case of an individual who enrolls under subsection (b)(2) in the month following the month in which the individual first satisfies subsection (a), the first day of the second month following the month in which the individual so enrolls.

(D) In the case of an individual who enrolls under subsection (b)(2) more than one month following the month in which the individual first satisfies subsection (a), the first day of the third month following the month in which the individual so enrolls.

(E) In the case of an individual who enrolls under subsection (b)(3), the July 1 following the month in which the individual so enrolls.

(2) An individual's coverage period under this section shall continue until the individual's enrollment is terminated as follows:

(A) As of the month following the month in which the Secretary provides notice to the individual that the individual no longer meets the condition described in subsection (a)(2)(B).

(B) As of the month following the month in which the individual files notice that the individual no longer wishes to participate in the insurance program established by this part.

(C) As of the month before the first month in which the individual becomes eligible for hospital insurance benefits under section 226 (a) or 226A.

(D) As of a date, determined under regulations of the Secretary, for non-payment of premiums.

The regulations under subparagraph (D) may provide a grace period of not longer than 90 days, which may be extended to not to exceed 180 days in any case where the Secretary determines that there was good cause for failure to pay the overdue premiums within such 90 day period. Termination of coverage under this section shall result in simultaneous termination of any coverage affected under any other part of this title.

(3) The provisions of subsections (h) and (i) of section 1837 apply to enrollment and nonenrollment under this section in the same manner as they apply to enrollment and nonenrollment and special enrollment periods under section 1818.

(d)(1)(A) Premiums for enrollment under this section shall be paid to the Secretary at such times, and in such manner, as the Secretary shall by regulations prescribe, and shall be deposited in the Treasury to the credit of the Federal Hospital Insurance Trust Fund.

(B)(i) Subject to clause (ii), such premiums shall be payable for the period commencing with the first month of an individual's coverage period and ending with the month in which the individual dies or, if earlier, in which the individual's coverage period terminates.

(ii) Such premiums shall not be payable for any month in which the individual is eligible for benefits under this part pursuant to section 226(b).

(2) The provisions of subsections (d) through (f) of section 1818 (relating to premiums) shall apply to individuals enrolled under this section in the same manner as they apply to individuals enrolled under that section.

PART B—SUPPLEMENTARY MEDICAL INSURANCE BENEFITS FOR THE AGED AND DISABLED[57]

Establishment of Supplementary Medical Insurance Program for the Aged and the Disabled

Sec. 1831. [42 U.S.C. 1395j] There is hereby established a voluntary insurance program to provide medical insurance benefits in accordance with the provisions of this part for aged and disabled individuals who elect to enroll under such program, to be financed from premium payments by enrollees together with contributions from funds appropriated by the Federal Government.

Scope of Benefits
Sec. 1832. [42 U.S.C. 1395k]

(a) The benefits provided to an individual by the insurance program established by this part shall consist of—
  (1) entitlement to have payment made to him or on his behalf (subject to the
  provisions of this part) for medical and other health services, except
  those described in subparagraphs (B) and (D) of paragraph (2) and subparagraphs (E) and (F) of section 1842(b)(6); and
  (2) entitlement to have pa yment made on his behalf (subject to the provisions of this part) for—
    (A) home health services (other than items described in subparagraph
      (G) or subparagraph (I));
    (B) medical and other health services (other than items described in sub-
      paragraph (G) or subparagraph (I)) furnished by a provider of serv-
      ices or by others under arrangement with them made by a provider
      of services, excluding—
        (i) physician services except where furnished by—
          (I) a resident or intern of a hospital, or
          (II) a physician to a patient in a hospital which has a teaching pro-
            gram approved as specified in paragraph (6) of section 1861(b)
            (including services in conjunction with the teaching programs
            of such hospital whether or not such patient is an inpatient of
            such hospital) where the conditions specified in paragraph (7)
            of such section are met,
        (ii) services for which payment may be made pursuant to section
          1835(b)(2),
        (iii) services described by section 1861(s)(2)(K)(i), certified nurse-
          midwife services, qualified psychologist services, and services of
          a certified registered nurse anesthetist;
        (iv) services of a nurse practitioner or clinical nurse specialist but
          only if no facility or other provider charges or is paid any amounts
          with respect to the furnishing of such services; and
    (C) outpatient physical therapy services (other than services to which
      the second sentence of section 1861(p) applies), outpatient[58] occu-
      pational therapy services (other than services to which such sentence
      applies through the operation of section 1861(g), and outpatient
      speech-language pathology services (other than services to which
      the second sentence of section 1861(p) applies through the applica-
      tion of section 1861(ll)(2))[59];
    (D)(i) rural health clinic services and (ii) Federally qualified health
      center services;
    (E) comprehensive outpatient rehabilitation facility services;
    (F) facility services furnished in connection with surgical procedures
      specified by the Secretary—
        (i) pursuant to section 1833(i)(1)(A) and performed in an ambulatory
          surgical center (which meets health, safety, and other standards

specified by the Secretary in regulations) if the center has an agreement in effect with the Secretary by which the center agrees to accept the standard overhead amount determined under section 1833(i)(2)(A) as full payment for such services (including intra-ocular lens in cases described in section 1833(i)(2)(A)(iii)) and to accept an assignment described in section 1842(b)(3)(B)(ii) with respect to payment for all such services (including intraocu-lar lens in cases described in section 1833(i)(2)(A)(iii)) furnished by the center to individuals enrolled under this part, or

(ii) pursuant to section 1833(i)(1)(B) and performed by a physician, described in paragraph (1), (2), or (3) of section 1861(r), in his office, if the Secretary has determined that—

    (I) a quality control and peer review organization (having a con-tract with the Secretary under part B of title XI of this Act) is willing, able, and has agreed to carry out a review (on a sample or other reasonable basis) of the physician's performing such procedures in the physician's office,

    (II) the particular physician involved has agreed to make available to such organization such records as the Secretary determines to be necessary to carry out the review, and

    (III) the physician is authorized to perform the procedure in a hos-pital located in the area in which the office is located,

      and if the physician agrees to accept the standard overhead amount determined under section 1833(i)(2)(B) as full payment for such services and to accept payment on an assignment-related basis with respect to payment for all services (including all pre-and post-operative services) described in paragraphs (1) and (2)(A) of section 1861(s) and furnished in connection with such surgical procedure to individuals enrolled under this part;

(G) covered items (described in section 1834(a)(13)) furnished by a pro-vider of services or by others under arrangements with them made by a provider of services;

(H) outpatient critical access hospital services (as defined in section 1861(mm)(3));

(I) prosthetic devices and orthotics and prosthetics (described in section 1834(h)(4)) furnished by a provider of services or by others under arrangements with them made by a provider of services; and

(J) partial hospitalization services provided by a community mental health center (as described in section 1861(ff)(2)(B)).

(b) For definitions of "spell of illness," "medical and other health services," and other terms used in this part, see section 1861.

Payment of Benefits[60]

Sec. 1833. [42 U.S.C. 1395l]

(a) Except as provided in section 1876, and subject to the succeeding provi-sions of this section, there shall be paid from the Federal Supplementary

Medical Insurance Trust Fund, in the case of each individual who is covered under the insurance program established by this part and incurs expenses for services with respect to which benefits are payable under this part, amounts equal to—

(1) in the case of services described in section 1832(a)(1)—80 percent of the reasonable charges for the services; except that (A) an organization which provides medical and other health services (or arranges for their availability) on a prepayment basis (and either is sponsored by a union or employer, or does not provide, or arrange for the provision of, any inpatient hospital services) may elect to be paid 80 percent of the reasonable cost of services for which payment may be made under this part on behalf of individuals enrolled in such organization in lieu of 80 percent of the reasonable charges for such services if the organization undertakes to charge such individuals no more than 20 percent of such reasonable cost plus any amounts payable by them as a result of subsection (b), (B) with respect to items and services described in section 1861 (s)(10)(A), the amounts paid shall be 100 percent of the reasonable charges for such items and services, (C) with respect to expenses incurred for those physicians' services for which payment may be made under this part that are described in section 1862(a)(4), the prosthetic devices and orthotics and prosthetics (as defined in section 1834(h) (4)), the amounts paid shall be the amounts described in section 1834 (h)(1), the amounts paid shall be subject to such limitations as may be prescribed by regulations, (D) with respect to clinical diagnostic laboratory tests for which payment is made under this part (i) on the basis of a fee schedule under subsection (h)(1) or section 1834(d)(1), the amount paid shall be equal to 80 percent (or 100 percent, in the case of such tests for which payment is made on an assignment-related basis) of the lesser of the amount determined under such fee schedule, the limitation amount for that test determined under subsection (h)(4)(B), or the amount of the charges billed for the tests, or (ii) on the basis of a negotiated rate established under subsection (h)(6), the amount paid shall be equal to 100 percent of such negotiated rate, (E) with respect to services furnished to individuals who have been determined to have end stage renal disease, the amounts paid shall be determined subject to the provisions of section 1881, (F) with respect to clinical social worker services under section 1861(s)(2)(N), the amounts paid shall be 80 percent of the lesser of (i) the actual charge for the services or (ii) 75 percent of the amount determined for payment of a psychologist under clause (L), (G) with respect to facility services furnished in connection with a surgical procedure specified pursuant to subsection (i) (1)(A) and furnished to an individual in an ambulatory surgical center described in such subsection, for services furnished beginning with the implementation date of a revised payment system for such services in such facilities specified in subsection (i)(2)(D), the amounts paid shall be 80 percent of the lesser of the actual charge for the services or the amount determined by the Secretary under such revised payment

system, (H) with respect to services of a certified registered nurse anesthetist under section 1861(s)(11), the amounts paid shall be 80 percent of the least of the actual charge, the prevailing charge that would be recognized (or, for services furnished on or after January 1, 1992, the fee schedule amount provided under section 1848) if the services had been performed by an anesthesiologist, or the fee schedule for such services established by the Secretary in accordance with subsection (1), (I) with respect to covered items (described in section 1834(a)(13)), the amounts paid shall be the amounts described in section 1834(a)(1), and (J) with respect to expenses incurred for radiologist services (as defined in section 1834(b)(6)), subject to section 1848, the amounts paid shall be 80 percent of the lesser of the actual charge for the services or the amount provided under the fee schedule established under section 1834(b), (K) with respect to certified nurse–midwife services under section 1861(s)(2)(L), the amounts paid shall be 80 percent of the lesser of the actual charge for the services or the amount determined by a fee schedule established by the Secretary for the purposes of this subparagraph (but in no event shall such fee schedule exceed 65 percent of the prevailing charge that would be allowed for the same service performed by a physician, or, for services furnished on or after January 1, 1992, 65 percent of the fee schedule amount provided under section 1848 for the same service performed by a physician), (L) with respect to qualified psychologist services under section 1861(s)(2)(M), the amounts paid shall be 80 percent of the lesser of the actual charge for the services or the amount determined by a fee schedule established by the Secretary for the purposes of this subparagraph, (M) with respect to prosthetic devices and orthotics and (N) with respect to expenses incurred for physicians' services (as defined in section 1848(j)(3)), the amounts paid shall be 80 percent of the payment basis determined under section 1848(a)(1), (O) with respect to services described in section 1861(s)(2)(K) (relating to services furnished by physicians assistants, nurse practitioners, or clinical nurse specialists), the amounts paid shall be equal to 80 percent of (i) the lesser of the actual charge or 85 percent of the fee schedule amount provided under section 1848, or (ii) in the case of services as an assistant at surgery, the lesser of the actual charge or 85 percent of the amount that would otherwise be recognized if performed by a physician who is serving as an assistant at surgery, (P) with respect to surgical dressings, the amounts paid shall be the amounts determined under section 1834(i), (Q) with respect to items or services for which fee schedules are established pursuant to section 1842(s), the amounts paid shall be 80 percent of the lesser of the actual charge or the fee schedule established in such section, (R) with respect to ambulance services, (i) the amounts paid shall be 80 percent of the lesser of the actual charge for the services or the amount determined by a fee schedule established by the Secretary under section 1834(l) and (ii) with respect to ambulance services described in section 1834 (l)(8), the amounts paid shall be the amounts determined under section

1834(g) for outpatient critical access hospital services, (S) with respect to drugs and biologicals (including intravenous immune globulin (as defined in section 1861(zz)) not paid on a cost or prospective payment basis as otherwise provided in this part (other than items and services described in subparagraph (B)), the amounts paid shall be 80 percent of the lesser of the actual charge or the payment amount established in section 1842(o) (or, if applicable, under section 1847, 1847A, or 1847B), (T) with respect to medical nutrition therapy services (as defined in section 1861(vv)), the amount paid shall be 80 percent of the lesser of the actual charge for the services or 85 percent of the amount determined under the fee schedule established under section 1848(b) for the same services if furnished by a physician, (U) with respect to facility fees described in section 1834(m)(2)(B), the amounts paid shall be 80 percent of the lesser of the actual charge or the amounts specified in such section, (V) notwithstanding subparagraphs (I) (relating to durable medical equipment), (M) (relating to prosthetic devices and orthotics and prosthetics), and (Q) (relating to 1842(s) items), with respect to competitively priced items and services (described in section 1847(a)(2)) that are furnished in a competitive area, the amounts paid shall be the amounts described in section 1847(b)(5), and (W) with respect to additional preventive services (as defined in section 1861 (ddd)(1)), the amount paid shall be (i) in the case of such services which are clinical diagnostic laboratory tests, the amount determined under subparagraph (D), and (ii) in the case of all other such services, 80 percent of the lesser of the actual charge for the service or the amount determined under a fee schedule established by the Secretary for purposes of this subparagraph;

(2) in the case of services described in section 1832(a)(2) (except those services described in subparagraphs (C), (D), (E), (F), (G), (H), and (I) of such section and unless otherwise specified in section 1881)—

   (A) with respect to home health services (other than a covered osteoporosis drug) (as defined in section 1861(kk)), the amount determined under the prospective payment system under section 1895;

   (B) with respect to other items and services (except those described in subparagraph (C), (D), or (E) of this paragraph and except as may be provided in section 1886 or section 1888(e)(9))—

      (i) furnished before January 1, 1999, the lesser of—

         (I) the reasonable cost of such services, as determined under section 1861(v), or

         (II) the customary charges with respect to such services,

            less the amount a provider may charge as described in clause (ii) of section 1866(a)(2)(A), but in no case may the payment for such other services exceed 80 percent of such reasonable cost, or

      (ii) if such services are furnished before January 1, 1999, by a public provider of services, or by another provider which demonstrates to the satisfaction of the Secretary that a significant portion of its patients are low-income (and requests that payment be made under this clause), free of charge or at nominal charges to the public, 80 percent of the amount determined in accordance with section 1814(b)(2), or

(iii) if such services are furnished on or after January 1, 1999, the amount determined under subsection (t), or

(iv) if (and for so long as) the conditions described in section 1814(b)(3) are met, the amounts determined under the reimbursement system described in such section;

(C) with respect to services described in the second sentence of section 1861(p), 80 percent of the reasonable charges for such services;

(D) with respect to clinical diagnostic laboratory tests for which payment is made under this part (i) on the basis of a fee schedule determined under subsection (h)(1) or section 1834(d)(1), the amount paid shall be equal to 80 percent (or 100 percent, in the case of such tests for which payment is made on an assignment-related basis or to a provider having an agreement under section 1866 of the lesser of the amount determined under such fee schedule, the limitation amount for that test determined under subsection (h)(4)(B), or the amount of the charges billed for the tests, (ii) on the basis of a negotiated rate established under subsection (h)(6), the amount paid shall be equal to 100 percent of such negotiated rate for such tests; or (iii) on the basis of a rate established under a demonstration project under section 1847(e), the amount paid shall be equal to 100 percent of such rate,

(E) with respect to—

(i) outpatient hospital radiology services (including diagnostic and therapeutic radiology, nuclear medicine and CAT scan procedures, magnetic resonance imaging, and ultrasound and other imaging services, but excluding screening mammography and, for services furnished on or after January 1, 2005, diagnostic mammography), and

(ii) effective for procedures performed on or after October 1, 1989, diagnostic procedures (as defined by the Secretary) described in section 1861(s)(3) (other than diagnostic x-ray tests and diagnostic laboratory tests),

the amount determined under subsection (n) or, for services or procedures performed on or after January 1, 1999, subsection (t);

(F) with respect to a covered osteoporosis drug (as defined in section 1861 (kk)) furnished by a home health agency, 80 percent of the reasonable cost of such service, as determined under section 1861(v); and

(G) with respect to items and services described in section 1861(s)(10)(A), the lesser of—

(i) the reasonable cost of such services, as determined under section 1861(v), or

(ii) the customary charges with respect to such services,

or, if such services are furnished by a public provider of services, or by another provider which demonstrates to the satisfaction of the Secretary that a significant portion of its patients are low-income (and requests that payment be made under this provision), free of charge or at nominal charges to the public, the amount determined in accordance with section 1814(b)(2);

(3) in the case of services described in section 1832(a)(2)(D)—

(A) except as provided in subparagraph (B), the costs which are reasonable and related to the cost of furnishing such services or which are based on such other tests of reasonableness as the Secretary may prescribe in regulations, including those authorized under section 1861 (v)(1)(A), less the amount a provider may charge as described in clause (ii) of section 1866(a)(2)(A), but in no case may the payment for such services (other than for items and services described in section 1861(s)(10)(A)) exceed 80 percent of such costs; or

(B) with respect to the services described in clause (ii) of section 1832 (a)(2)(D) that are furnished to an individual enrolled with a MA plan under part C pursuant to a written agreement described in section 1853(a)(4), the amount (if any) by which—

(i) the amount of payment that would have otherwise been provided under subparagraph (A) (calculated as if "100 percent" were substituted for "80 percent" in such subparagraph) for such services if the individual had not been so enrolled; exceeds

(ii) the amount of the payments received under such written agreement for such services (not including any financial incentives provided for in such agreement such as risk pool payments, bonuses, or withholds), less the amount the federally qualified health center may charge as described in section 1857(e)(3)(B);

REST of Section 1833 is not included nor is Section 1834.

Procedure for Payment of Claims of Providers of Services
Sec. 1835. [42 U.S.C. 1395n]

(a) Except as provided in subsections (b), (c), and (e), payment for services described in section 1832(a)(2) furnished an individual may be made only to providers of services which are eligible therefor under section 1866(a), and only if—

(1) written request, signed by such individual, except in cases in which the Secretary finds it impracticable for the individual to do so, is filed for such payment in such form, in such manner and by such person or persons as the Secretary may by regulation prescribe, no later than the close of the period of 3 calendar years following the year in which such services are furnished (deeming any services furnished in the last 3 calendar months of any calendar year to have been furnished in the succeeding calendar year) except that, where the Secretary deems that efficient administration so requires, such period may be reduced to not less than 1 calendar year; and

(2) a physician certifies (and recertifies, where such services are furnished over a period of time, in such cases, with such frequency, and accompanied by such supporting material, appropriate to the case involved, as may be provided by regulations) that—

   (A) in the case of home health services (i) such services are or were required because the individual is or was confined to his home (except when receiving items and services referred to in section 1861(m)(7)) and needs or needed skilled nursing care (other than solely venipuncture for the purpose of obtaining a blood sample) on an intermittent basis or physical or speech therapy or, in the case of an individual who has been furnished home health services based on such a need and who no longer has such a need for such care or therapy, continues or continued to need occupational therapy, (ii) a plan for furnishing such services to such individual has been established and is periodically reviewed by a physician, and (iii) such services are or were furnished while the individual is or was under the care of a physician;

   (B) in the case of medical and other health services, except services described in subparagraphs (B), (C), and (D) of section 1861(s)(2), such services are or were medically required;

   (C) in the case of outpatient physical therapy services or outpatient occupational therapy services, (i) such services are or were required because the individual needed physical therapy services or occupational therapy services, respectively, (ii) a plan for furnishing such services has been established by a physician or by the qualified physical therapist or qualified occupational therapist, respectively, providing such services and is periodically reviewed by a physician, and (iii) such services are or were furnished while the individual is or was under the care of a physician;

   (D) in the case of outpatient speech pathology services, (i) such services are or were required because the individual needed speech pathology services, (ii) a plan for furnishing such services has been established by a physician or by the speech pathologist providing such services and is periodically reviewed by a physician, and (iii) such services are or were furnished while the individual is or was under the care of a physician;

   (E) in the case of comprehensive outpatient rehabilitation facility services, (i) such services are or were required because the individual needed skilled rehabilitation services, (ii) a plan for furnishing such services has been established and is periodically reviewed by a physician, and (iii) such services are or were furnished while the individual is or was under the care of a physician; and

   (F) in the case of partial hospitalization services, (i) the individual would require inpatient psychiatric care in the absence of such services, (ii) an individualized, written plan for furnishing such services has been established by a physician and is reviewed periodically by a physician, and (iii) such services are or were furnished while the individual is or was under the care of a physician.

For purposes of this section, the term "provider of services" shall include a clinic, rehabilitation agency, or public health agency if, in the case of a clinic or rehabilitation agency, such clinic or agency meets the requirements of section 1861(p)(4)(A) (or meets the requirements of such section through the operation of section 1861(g)[145]), or if, in the case of a public health agency, such agency meets the requirements of section 1861 (p)(4)(B) (or meets the requirements of such section through the operation of section 1861(g)[146]), but only with respect to the furnishing of outpatient physical therapy services[147] (as therein defined) or (through the operation of section 1861(g)[148]) with respect to the furnishing of outpatient occupational therapy services.

To the extent provided by regulations, the certification and recertification requirements of paragraph (2) shall be deemed satisfied where, at a later date, a physician makes a certification of the kind provided in subparagraph (A) or (B) of paragraph (2) (whichever would have applied), but only where such certification is accompanied by such medical and other evidence as may be required by such regulations. With respect to the physician certification required by paragraph (2) for home health services furnished to any individual by a home health agency (other than an agency which is a governmental entity) and with respect to the establishment and review of a plan for such services, the Secretary shall prescribe regulations which shall become effective no later than July 1, 1981, and which prohibit a physician who has a significant ownership interest in, or a significant financial or contractual relationship with, such home health agency from performing such certification and from establishing or reviewing such plan, except that such prohibition shall not apply with respect to a home health agency which is a sole community home health agency (as determined by the Secretary). For purposes of the preceding sentence, service by a physician as an uncompensated officer or director of a home health agency shall not constitute having a significant ownership interest in, or a significant financial or contractual relationship with, such agency. For purposes of paragraph (2)(A), an individual shall be considered to be "confined to his home" if the individual has a condition, due to an illness or injury, that restricts the ability of the individual to leave his or her home except with the assistance of another individual or the aid of a supportive device (such as crutches, a cane, a wheelchair, or a walker), or if the individual has a condition such that leaving his or her home is medically contraindicated. While an individual does not have to be bedridden to be considered "confined to his home," the condition of the individual should be such that there exists a normal inability to leave home and that leaving home requires a considerable and taxing effort by the individual. Any absence of an individual from the home attributable to the need to receive health care treatment, including regular absences for the purpose of participating in therapeutic, psychosocial, or medical treatment in an adult day-care program that is licensed or certified by a State, or accredited, to furnish adult day-care services in the State shall not disqualify an individual from being considered to be "confined to his home." Any other absence of an individual from the home shall not so disqualify an individual if the absence is of infrequent or of relatively short duration. For purposes of the preceding sentence, any absence for the purpose of attending a religious service shall be deemed to be an absence of infrequent or short duration.

(b)(1) Payment may also be made to any hospital for services described in section 1861(s) furnished as an outpatient service by a hospital or by others under arrangements made by it to an individual entitled to benefits under this part even though such hospital does not have an agreement in effect under this title if (A) such services were emergency services, (B) the Secretary would be required to make such payment if the hospital had such an agreement in effect and otherwise met the conditions of payment hereunder, and (C) such hospital has made an election pursuant to section 1814(d)(1)(C) with respect to the calendar year in which such emergency services are provided. Such payments shall be made only in the amounts provided under section 1833(a)(2) and then only if such hospital agrees to comply, with respect to the emergency services provided, with the provisions of section 1866(a).

(2) Payment may also be made on the basis of an itemized bill to an individual for services described in paragraph (1) of this subsection if (A) payment cannot be made under such paragraph (1) solely because the hospital does not elect, in accordance with section 1814(d)(1)(C), to claim such payments and (B) such individual files application (submitted within such time and in such form and manner, and containing and supported by such information as the Secretary shall by regulations prescribe) for reimbursement. The amounts payable under this paragraph shall, subject to the provisions of section 1833, be equal to 80 percent of the hospital's reasonable charges for such services.

(c) Notwithstanding the provisions of this section and sections 1832, 1833, and 1866(a)(1)(A), a hospital or a critical access hospital may, subject to such limitations as may be prescribed by regulations, collect from an individual the customary charges for services specified in section 1861 (s) and furnished to him by such hospital as an outpatient, but only if such charges for such services do not exceed the applicable supplementary medical insurance deductible, and such customary charges shall be regarded as expenses incurred by such individual with respect to which benefits are payable in accordance with section 1833(a)(1). Payments under this title to hospitals which have elected to make collections from individuals in accordance with the preceding sentence shall be adjusted periodically to place the hospital in the same position it would have been had it instead been reimbursed in accordance with section 1833(a) (2) (or, in the case of a critical access hospital, in accordance with section 1833(a)(6)).

(d) Subject to section 1880, no payment may be made under this part to any Federal provider of services or other Federal agency, except a provider of services which the Secretary determines is providing services to the public generally as a community institution or agency; and no such payment may be made to any provider of services or other person for any item or service which such provider or person is obligated by a law of, or a contract with, the United States to render at public expense.

(e) For purposes of services (1) which are inpatient hospital services by reason of paragraph (7) of section 1861(b) or for which entitlement exists by reason of clause (II) of section 1832(a)(2)(B)(i), and (2) for which the reasonable cost thereof is determined under section 1861(v)(1)(D) (or would be if section 1886 did not apply), payment under this part shall be made to such fund as may be designated by the organized medical staff of the hospital in which such services were furnished or, if such services were furnished in such hospital by the faculty of a medical school, to such fund as may be designated by such faculty, but only if—

(A) such hospital has an agreement with the Secretary under section 1866, and

(B) the Secretary has received written assurances that (i) such payment will be used by such fund solely for the improvement of care to patients in such hospital or for educational or charitable purposes and (ii) the individuals who were furnished such services or any other persons will not be charged for such services (or if charged provision will be made for return of any moneys incorrectly collected).

Eligible Individuals

Sec. 1836. [42 U.S.C. 1395o] Every individual who—

(1) is entitled to hospital insurance benefits under part A, or
(2) has attained age 65 and is a resident of the United States, and is either (A) a citizen or (B) an alien lawfully admitted for permanent residence who has resided in the United States continuously during the 5 years immediately preceding the month in which he applies for enrollment under this part, is eligible to enroll in the insurance program established by this part.

Amounts of Premiums

Sec. 1839. [42 U.S.C. 1395r]

(a)(1) The Secretary shall, during September of 1983 and of each year thereafter, determine the monthly actuarial rate for enrollees age 65 and over which shall be applicable for the succeeding calendar year. Such actuarial rate shall be the amount the Secretary estimates to be necessary so that the aggregate amount for such calendar year with respect to those enrollees age 65 and older will equal one-half of the total of the benefits and administrative costs which he estimates will be payable from the Federal Supplementary Medical Insurance Trust Fund for services performed and related administrative costs incurred in such calendar year with respect to such enrollees. In calculating the monthly actuarial rate, the Secretary shall include an appropriate amount for a contingency margin.

(2) The monthly premium of each individual enrolled under this part for each month after December 1983 shall be the amount determined under paragraph (3). adjusted as required in accordance with subsections (b), (c), (f), and (i) of this section, and to reflect any credit provided under section 1854(b)(1)(C)(ii)(III).

(3) The Secretary, during September of each year, shall determine and promulgate a monthly premium rate for the succeeding calendar year that (except as provided in subsection (g)) is equal to 50 percent of the monthly actuarial rate for enrollees age 65 and over, determined according to paragraph (1), for that succeeding calendar year.

Whenever the Secretary promulgates the dollar amount which shall be applicable as the monthly premium rate for any period, he shall, at the time such promulgation is announced, issue a public statement setting forth the actuarial assumptions and bases employed by him in arriving at the amount of an adequate actuarial rate for enrollees age 65 and older as provided in paragraph (1).

(4) The Secretary shall also, during September of 1983 and of each year thereafter, determine the monthly actuarial rate for disabled enrollees under age 65 which shall be applicable for the succeeding calendar year. Such actuarial rate shall be the amount the Secretary estimates to be necessary so that the aggregate amount for such calendar year with respect to disabled enrollees under age 65 will equal one-half of the total of the benefits and administrative costs which he estimates will be payable from the Federal Supplementary Medical Insurance Trust Fund for services performed and related administrative costs incurred in such calendar year with respect to such enrollees. In calculating the monthly actuarial rate under this paragraph, the Secretary shall include an appropriate amount for a contingency margin.

(b) In the case of an individual whose coverage period began pursuant to an enrollment after his initial enrollment period (determined pursuant to subsection (c) or (d) of section 1837) and not pursuant to a special enrollment period under section 1837(i)(4), the monthly premium determined under subsection (a) (without regard to any adjustment under subsection (i)) shall be increased by 10 percent of the monthly premium so determined for each full 12 months (in the same continuous period of eligibility) in which he could have been but was not enrolled. For purposes of the preceding sentence, there shall be taken into account (1) the months which elapsed between the close of his initial enrollment period and the close of the enrollment period in which he enrolled, plus (in the case of an individual who reenrolls) (2) the months which elapsed between the date of termination of a previous coverage period and the close of the enrollment period in which he reenrolled, but there shall not be taken into account months for which the individual can demonstrate that the individual was enrolled in a group health plan described in section 1862(b)(1)(A)(v) by reason of the individual's (or the individual's spouse's) current employment status or months during which the individual has not attained the age of 65 and for which the individual can demonstrate that the individual was enrolled in a large group health plan (as that term is defined in section 1862(b)(1)(B) (iii)) by reason of the individual's current employment status (or the current employment status of a family member of the individual) or months for which the individual can demonstrate that the individual was and individual described in section 1837(k)(3). Any increase in an individual's monthly premium under the first sentence of this subsection with respect to a particular continuous period of eligibility shall not be applicable with respect to any other continuous period of eligibility which such individual may have. No increase in the premium shall be effected for a month in the case of an individual who enrolls under this part during 2001, 2002, 2003, or 2004 and who demonstrates to the Secretary before December 31, 2004, that the individual is a covered beneficiary (as defined in section 1072(5) of title 10, United States Code). The Secretary of Health and Human Services shall consult with the Secretary of Defense in identifying individuals described in the previous sentence.

(c) If any monthly premium determined under the foregoing provisions of this section is not a multiple of 10 cents, such premium shall be rounded to the nearest multiple of 10 cents.

(d) For purposes of subsection (b) (and section 1837(g)(1)), an individual's "continuous period of eligibility" is the period beginning with the first day on which he is eligible to enroll under section 1836 and ending with his death; except that any period during all of which an individual satisfied paragraph (1) of section 1836 and which terminated in or before the month preceding the month in which he attained age 65 shall be a separate "continuous period of eligibility" with respect to such individual (and each such period which terminates shall be deemed not to have existed for purposes of subsequently applying this section).

(e)(1) Upon the request of a State (or any appropriate State or local governmental entity specified by the Secretary), the Secretary may enter into an agreement with the State (or such entity) under which the State (or such entity) agrees to pay on a quarterly or other periodic basis to the Secretary (to be deposited in the Treasury to the credit of the Federal Supplementary Medical Insurance Trust Fund) an amount equal to the amount of the part B late enrollment premium increases with respect to the premiums for eligible individuals (as defined in paragraph (3)(A)).

(2) No part B late enrollment premium increase shall apply to an eligible individual for premiums for months for which the amount of such an increase is payable under an agreement under paragraph (1).

(3) In this subsection:

(A) The term "eligible individual" means an individual who is enrolled under this part B and who is within a class of individuals specified in the agreement under paragraph (1).

(B) The term "part B late enrollment premium increase" means any increase in a premium as a result of the application of subsection (b).

(f) For any calendar year after 1988, if an individual is entitled to monthly benefits under section 202 or 223 or to a monthly annuity under section 3 (a), 4(a), or 4(f) of the Railroad Retirement Act of 1974[153] for November and December of the preceding year, if the monthly premium of the individual under this section for December and for January is deducted from those benefits under section 1840(a)(1) or section 1840(b)(1), and if the amount of the individual's premium is not adjusted for such January under subsection (i), the monthly premium otherwise determined under this section for an individual for that year shall not be increased, pursuant to this subsection, to the extent that such increase would reduce the amount of benefits payable to that individual for that December below the amount of benefits payable to that individual for that November (after the deduction of the premium under this section). For purposes of this subsection, retroactive adjustments or payments and deductions on account of work shall not be taken into account in determining the monthly benefits to which an individual is entitled under section 202 or 223 or under the Railroad Retirement Act of 1974.

(g) In estimating the benefits and administrative costs which will be payable from the Federal Supplementary Medical Insurance Trust Fund for a year for purposes of determining the monthly premium rate under subsection (a)(3), the Secretary shall exclude an estimate of any benefits and administrative costs attributable to—

  (1) the application of section 1861(v)(1)(L)(viii) or to the establishment under section 1861(v)(1)(L)(i)(V) of a per visit limit at 106 percent of the median (instead of 105 percent of the median), but only to the extent payment for home health services under this title is not being made under section 1895 (relating to prospective payment for home health services); and

  (2) the medicare prescription drug discount card and transitional assistance program under section 1860D-31

(h) Potential Application of Comparative Cost Adjustment in CCA Areas.—

  (1) In general.—Certain individuals who are residing in a CCA area under section 1860C-1 who are not enrolled in an MA plan under part C may be subject to a premium adjustment under subsection (f) of such section for months in which the CCA program under such section is in effect in such area.

  (2) No effect on late enrollment penalty or income-related adjustment in subsidies.—Nothing in this subsection or section 1860C-1(f) shall be construed as affecting the amount of any premium adjustment under subsection (b) or (i). Subsection (f) shall be applied without regard to any premium adjustment referred to in paragraph (1).

  (3) Implementation.—In order to carry out a premium adjustment under this subsection and section 1860C-1(f) (insofar as it is effected through the manner of collection of premiums under section 1840(a)), the Secretary shall transmit to the Commissioner of Social Security—

    (A) at the beginning of each year, the name, social security account number, and the amount of the premium adjustment (if any) for each individual enrolled under this part for each month during the year; and

(B) periodically throughout the year, information to update the information previously transmitted under this paragraph for the year.

(i) Reduction in Premium Subsidy Based on Income.—

(1) In general.—In the case of an individual whose modified adjusted gross income exceeds the threshold amount under paragraph (2), the monthly amount of the premium subsidy applicable to the premium under this section for a month after December 2006 shall be reduced (and the monthly premium shall be increased) by the monthly adjustment amount specified in paragraph (3).

(2) Threshold amount.—For purposes of this subsection, the threshold amount is—

(A) except as provided in subparagraph (B), $80,000, and

(B) in the case of a joint return, twice the amount applicable under subparagraph (A) for the calendar year.

(3) Monthly adjustment amount.—

(A) In general.—Subject to subparagraph (B), the monthly adjustment amount specified in this paragraph for an individual for a month in a year is equal to the product of the following:

(i) Sliding scale percentage.—The applicable percentage specified in the table in subparagraph (C) for the individual minus 25 percentage points.

(ii) Unsubsidized part b premium amount.—200 percent of the monthly actuarial rate for enrollees age 65 and over (as determined under subsection (a)(1) for the year).

(B) 3-year phase in.—The monthly adjustment amount specified in this paragraph for an individual for a month in a year before 2009 is equal to the following percentage of the monthly adjustment amount specified in subparagraph (A):

(i) For 2007, 33 percent.

(ii) For 2008, 67 percent.

(C) Applicable percentage.—

(i) In general.—

If the modified adjusted gross is:	The applicable percentage is:
More than $80,000 but not more than $100,000	35 percent
More than $100,000 but not more than $150,000	50 percent
More than $150,000 but not more than $200,000	65 percent
More than $200,000	80 percent.

(ii) Joint returns.—In the case of a joint return, clause (i) shall be applied by substituting dollar amounts which are twice the dollar amounts otherwise applicable under clause (i) for the calendar year.

(iii) Married individuals filing separate returns.—In the case of an individual who—

(I) is married as of the close of the taxable year (within the meaning of section 7703 of the Internal Revenue Code of 1986) but does not file a joint return for such year, and

(II) does not live apart from such individual's spouse at all times during the taxable year, clause (i) shall be applied by reducing each of the dollar amounts otherwise applicable under such clause for the calendar year by the threshold amount for such year applicable to an unmarried individual.

(4) Modified adjusted gross income.—

(A) In general.—For purposes of this subsection, the term "modified adjusted gross income" means adjusted gross income (as defined in section 62 of the Internal Revenue Code of 1986)—

(i) determined without regard to sections 135, 911, 931, and 933 of such Code; and

(ii) increased by the amount of interest received or accrued during the taxable year which is exempt from tax under such Code. In the case of an individual filing a joint return, any reference in this subsection to the modified adjusted gross income of such individual shall be to such return's modified adjusted gross income.

(B) Taxable year to be used in determining modified adjusted gross income.—

(i) In general.—In applying this subsection for an individual's premiums in a month in a year, subject to clause (ii) and subparagraph (C), the individual's modified adjusted gross income shall be such income determined for the individual's last taxable year beginning in the second calendar year preceding the year involved.

(ii) Temporary use of other data.—If, as of October 15 before a calendar year, the Secretary of the Treasury does not have adequate data for an individual in appropriate electronic form for the taxable year referred to in clause (i), the individual's modified adjusted gross income shall be determined using the data in such form from the previous taxable year. Except as provided in regulations prescribed by the Commissioner of Social Security in consultation with the Secretary, the preceding sentence shall cease to apply when adequate data in appropriate electronic form are available for the individual for the taxable year referred to in clause (i), and proper adjustments shall be made to the extent that the premium adjustments determined under the preceding sentence were inconsistent with those determined using such taxable year.

(iii) Non-filers.—In the case of individuals with respect to whom the Secretary of the Treasury does not have adequate data in appropriate electronic form for either taxable year referred to in clause (i) or clause (ii), the Commissioner of Social Security, in consultation with the Secretary, shall prescribe regulations which provide for the treatment of the premium adjustment with respect to such individual under this subsection, including regulations which provide for—

(I) the application of the highest applicable percentage under paragraph (3)(C) to such individual if the Commissioner has information which indicates that such individual's modified adjusted gross income might exceed the threshold amount for the taxable year referred to in clause (i), and

(II) proper adjustments in the case of the application of an applicable percentage under subclause (I) to such individual which is inconsistent with such individual's modified adjusted gross income for such taxable year.

(C) Use of more recent taxable year.—

(i) In general.—The Commissioner of Social Security in consultation with the Secretary of the Treasury shall establish a procedures under which an individual's modified adjusted gross income shall, at the request of such individual, be determined under this subsection—

(I) for a more recent taxable year than the taxable year otherwise used under subparagraph (B), or

(II) by such methodology as the Commissioner, in consultation with such Secretary, determines to be appropriate, which may include a methodology for aggregating or disaggregating information from tax returns in the case of marriage or divorce.

(ii) Standard for granting requests.—A request under clause (i)(I) to use a more recent taxable year may be granted only if—

(I) the individual furnishes to such Commissioner with respect to such year such documentation, such as a copy of a filed Federal income tax return or an equivalent document, as the Commissioner specifies for purposes of determining the premium adjustment (if any) under this subsection; and

(II) the individual's modified adjusted gross income for such year is significantly less than such income for the taxable year determined under subparagraph (B) by reason of the death of such individual's spouse, the marriage or divorce of such individual, or other major life changing events specified in regulations prescribed by the Commissioner in consultation with the Secretary.

(5) Inflation adjustment.—

(A) In general.—In the case of any calendar year beginning after 2007, each dollar amount in paragraph (2) or (3) shall be increased by an amount equal to—

(i) such dollar amount, multiplied by

(ii) the percentage (if any) by which the average of the Consumer Price Index for all urban consumers (United States city average)

for the 12-month period ending with August of the preceding calendar year exceeds such average for the 12-month period ending
with August 2006.
    (B) Rounding.—If any dollar amount after being increased under sub-
paragraph (A) is not a multiple of $1,000, such dollar amount shall
be rounded to the nearest multiple of $1,000.
  (6) Joint return defined.—For purposes of this subsection, the term "joint
return" has the meaning given to such term by section 7701(a)(38) of
the Internal Revenue Code of 1986[154].

State Agreements for Coverage of Eligible Individuals Who are Receiving Money Payments Under Public Assistance Programs or are Eligible for Medical Assistance

Sec. 1843. [42 U.S.C. 1395v]

(a) The Secretary shall, at the request of a State made before January 1, 1970,
or during 1981 or after 1988, enter into an agreement with such State pursuant to which all eligible individuals in either of the coverage groups
described in subsection (b) (as specified in the agreement) will be enrolled
under the program established by this part.
(b) An agreement entered into with any State pursuant to subsection (a) may
be applicable to either of the following coverage groups:
  (1) individuals receiving money payments under the plan of such State
approved under title I or title XVI; or
  (2) individuals receiving money payments under all of the plans of such
State approved under titles I, X, XIV, and XVI, and part A of title IV.

Except as provided in subsection (g), there shall be excluded from any
coverage group any individual who is entitled to monthly insurance
benefits under title II or who is entitled to receive an annuity under the
Railroad Retirement Act of 1974[190]. Effective January 1, 1974, and subject to section 1902(f), the Secretary shall, at the request of any State not
eligible to participate in the State plan program established under title
XVI, continue in effect the agreement entered into under this
section with such State subject to such modifications as the Secretary
may by regulations provide to take account of the termination of any plans
of such State approved under titles I, X, XIV, and XVI and the establishment of the supplemental security income program under title XVI.
  (c) For purposes of this section, an individual shall be treated as an eligible
individual only if he is an eligible individual (within the meaning of section 1836) on the date an agreement covering him is entered into under
subsection (a) or he becomes an eligible individual (within the meaning
of such section) at any time after such date; and he shall be treated as
receiving money payments described in subsection (b) if he receives such
payments for the month in which the agreement is entered into or any
month thereafter.

(d) In the case of any individual enrolled pursuant to this section—

    (1) the monthly premium to be paid by the State shall be determined under section 1839 (without any increase under subsection (b) thereof);

    (2) his coverage period shall begin on whichever of the following is the latest:

        (A) July 1, 1966;

        (B) the first day of the third month following the month in which the State agreement is entered into;

        (C) the first day of the first month in which he is both an eligible individual and a member of a coverage group specified in the agreement under this section; or

        (D) such date as may be specified in the agreement; and

    (3) his coverage period attributable to the agreement with the State under this section shall end on the last day of whichever of the following first occurs:

        (A) the month in which he is determined by the State agency to have become ineligible both for money payments of a kind specified in the agreement and (if there is in effect a modification entered into under subsection (h)) for medical assistance, or

        (B) the month preceding the first month for which he becomes entitled to monthly benefits under title II or to an annuity or pension under the Railroad Retirement Act of 1974.

(e) Any individual whose coverage period attributable to the State agreement is terminated pursuant to subsection (d)(3) shall be deemed for purposes of this part (including the continuation of his coverage period under this part) to have enrolled under section 1837 in the initial general enrollment period provided by section 1837(c). The coverage period under this part of any such individual who (in the last month of his coverage period attributable to the State agreement or in any of the following six months) files notice that he no longer wishes to participate in the insurance program established by this part, shall terminate at the close of the month in which the notice is filed.

(f) With respect to eligible individuals receiving money payments under the plan of a State approved under title I, X, XIV, or XVI, or part A of title IV, or eligible to receive medical assistance under the plan of such State approved under title XIX, if the agreement entered into under this section so provides, the term "carrier" as defined in section 1842(f) also includes the State agency, specified in such agreement, which administers or supervises the administration of the plan of such State approved under title I, XVI, or XIX. The agreement shall also contain such provisions as will facilitate the financial transactions of the State and the carrier with respect to deductions, coinsurance, and otherwise, and as will lead to economy and efficiency of operation, with respect to individuals receiving money payments under plans of the State approved under titles I, X, XIV, and XVI, and part A of title IV, and individuals eligible to receive medical assistance under the plan of the State approved under title XIX.

(g)(1) The Secretary shall, at the request of a State made before January 1, 1970, or during 1981 or after 1988, enter into a modification of an agreement entered into with such State pursuant to subsection (a) under which the second sentence of subsection (b) shall not apply with respect to such agreement.

(2) In the case of any individual who would (but for this subsection) be excluded from the applicable coverage group described in subsection (b) by the second sentence of such subsection—

(A) subsections (c) and (d)(2) shall be applied as if such subsections referred to the modification under this subsection (in lieu of the agreement under subsection (a)), and

(B) subsection (d)(3)(B) shall not apply so long as there is in effect a modification entered into by the State under this subsection.

(h)(1) The Secretary shall, at the request of a State made before January 1, 1970, or during 1981 or after 1988, enter into a modification of an agreement entered into with such State pursuant to subsection (a) under which the coverage group described in subsection (b) and specified in such agreement is broadened to include (A) individuals who are eligible to receive medical assistance under the plan of such State approved under title XIX, or (B) qualified medicare beneficiaries (as defined in section 1905(p)(1)).

(2) For purposes of this section, an individual shall be treated as eligible to receive medical assistance under the plan of the State approved under title XIX if, for the month in which the modification is entered into under this subsection or for any month thereafter, he has been determined to be eligible to receive medical assistance under such plan. In the case of any individual who would (but for this subsection) be excluded from the agreement, subsections (c) and (d)(2) shall be applied as if they referred to the modification under this subsection (in lieu of the agreement under subsection (a)), and subsection (d)(2)(C) shall be applied (except in the case of qualified medicare beneficiaries, as defined in section 1905(p)(1)) by substituting "second month following the first month" for "first month."

(3) In this subsection, the term "qualified medicare beneficiary" also includes an individual described in section 1902(a)(10)(E)(iii).

(i) For provisions relating to enrollment of qualified medicare beneficiaries under part A, see section 1818(g).

Payment for Physicians' Services[227]

Sec. 1848. [42 U.S.C. 1395w–4]

(a) Payment Based on Fee Schedule.—

(1) In general.—Effective for all physicians' services (as defined in subsection (j)(3)) furnished under this part during a year (beginning with 1992) for which payment is otherwise made on the basis of a reasonable charge or on the basis of a fee schedule under section 1834(b), payment under this part shall instead be based on the lesser of—

(A) the actual charge for the service, or

(B) subject to the succeeding provisions of this subsection, the amount determined under the fee schedule established under subsection (b) for services furnished during that year (in this subsection referred to as the "fee schedule amount").

Only Part 1 of Section 1848 on Payment for Physician Services is included.

PART C—MEDICARE + CHOICE PROGRAM[314]

Eligibility, Election, and Enrollment

Sec. 1851. [42 U.S.C. 1395w–21]

(a) Choice of medicare benefits through medicare + choice plans.—
    (1) In general.—Subject to the provisions of this section, each Medicare + Choice eligible individual (as defined in paragraph (3)) is entitled to elect to receive benefits (other than qualified prescription drug benefits) under this title—
        (A) through the original medicare fee-for-service program under parts A and B, or
        (B) through enrollment in a Medicare + Choice plan under this part,

and may elect qualified prescription drug coverage in accordance with section 1860D-1.

    (2) Types of medicare + choice plans that may be available.—A Medicare + Choice plan may be any of the following types of plans of health insurance:
        (A) Coordinated care plans (including regional plans).—
            (i) In general.—Coordinated care plans which provide health care services, including but not limited to health maintenance organization plans (with or without point of service options), plans offered by provider-sponsored organizations (as defined in section 1855(d)), and regional or local preferred provider organization plans (including MA regional plans).
            (ii) Specialized ma plans for special needs individuals.—Specialized MA plans for special needs individuals (as defined in section 1859 (b)(6)) may be any type of coordinated care plan.
        (B) Combination of msa plan and contributions to medicare + choice msa.—An MSA plan, as defined in section 1859(b)(3), and a contribution into a Medicare + Choice medical savings account (MSA).
        (C) Private fee–for–service plans.—A Medicare + Choice private fee-for-service plan, as defined in section 1859(b)(2).
    (3) Medicare + choice eligible individual.—
        (A) In general.—In this title, subject to subparagraph (B), the term Medicare + Choice eligible individual means an individual who is entitled to benefits under part A and enrolled under part B.
        (B) Special rule for end-stage renal disease.—Such term shall not include an individual medically determined to have end-stage renal disease, except that—

        (i) an individual who develops end-stage renal disease while enrolled in a Medicare + Choice plan may continue to be enrolled in that plan; and

        (ii) in the case of such an individual who is enrolled in a Medicare + Choice plan under clause (i) (or subsequently under this clause), if the enrollment is discontinued under circumstances described in subsection (e)(4)(A), then the individual will be treated as a "Medicare + Choice eligible individual" for purposes of electing to continue enrollment in another Medicare + Choice plan.

(b) Special Rules.—

  (1) Residence requirement.—

    (A) In general.—Except as the Secretary may otherwise provide and except as provided in subparagraph (C), an individual is eligible to elect a Medicare + Choice plan offered by a Medicare + Choice organization only if the plan serves the geographic area in which the individual resides.

    (B) Continuation of enrollment permitted.—Pursuant to rules specified by the Secretary, the Secretary shall provide that an MA local plan may offer to all individuals residing in a geographic area the option to continue enrollment in the plan, notwithstanding that the individual no longer resides in the service area of the plan, so long as the plan provides that individuals exercising this option have, as part of the benefits under the original medicare fee-for-service program option, reasonable access within that geographic area to the full range of basic benefits, subject to reasonable cost sharing liability in obtaining such benefits.

    (C) Continuation of enrollment permitted where service changed.—Notwithstanding subparagraph (A) and in addition to subparagraph (B), if a Medicare + Choice organization eliminates from its service area a Medicare + Choice payment area that was previously within its service area, the organization may elect to offer individuals residing in all or portions of the affected area who would otherwise be ineligible to continue enrollment the option to continue enrollment in an MA local plan it offers so long as—

      (i) the enrollee agrees to receive the full range of basic benefits (excluding emergency and urgently needed care) exclusively at facilities designated by the organization within the plan service area; and

      (ii) there is no other Medicare + Choice plan offered in the area in which the enrollee resides at the time of the organization's election.

  (2) Special rule for certain individuals covered under FEHBP or eligible for veterans or military health benefits, veterans.—

    (A) FEHBP.—An individual who is enrolled in a health benefit plan under chapter 89 of title 5, United States Code, is not eligible to enroll in an MSA plan until such time as the Director of the Office of Management and Budget certifies to the Secretary that the Office of Personnel Management has adopted policies which will ensure that the enrollment of such individuals in such plans will not result in increased expenditures for the Federal Government for health benefit plans under such chapter.

(B) VA and DOD.—The Secretary may apply rules similar to the rules described in subparagraph (A) in the case of individuals who are eligible for health care benefits under chapter 55 of title 10, United States Code, or under chapter 17 of title 38 of such Code.

(3) Limitation on eligibility of qualified medicare beneficiaries and other medicaid beneficiaries to enroll in an msa plan.—An individual who is a qualified medicare beneficiary (as defined in section 1905(p)(1)), a qualified disabled and working individual (described in section 1905 (s)), an individual described in section 1902(a)(10)(E)(iii), or otherwise entitled to medicare cost-sharing under a State plan under title XIX is not eligible to enroll in an MSA plan.

(4) Coverage under MSA plans.—

(A) In general.—Under rules established by the Secretary, an individual is not eligible to enroll (or continue enrollment) in an MSA plan for a year unless the individual provides assurances satisfactory to the Secretary that the individual will reside in the United States for at least 183 days during the year.

(B) Evaluation.—The Secretary shall regularly evaluate the impact of permitting enrollment in MSA plans under this part on selection (including adverse selection), use of preventive care, access to care, and the financial status of the Trust Funds under this title.

(C) Reports.—The Secretary shall submit to Congress periodic reports on the numbers of individuals enrolled in such plans and on the evaluation being conducted under subparagraph (B).

(c) Process for Exercising Choice.—

(1) In general.—The Secretary shall establish a process through which elections described in subsection (a) are made and changed, including the form and manner in which such elections are made and changed. Such elections shall be made or changed only during coverage election periods specified under subsection (e) and shall become effective as provided in subsection (f).

(2) Coordination through medicare + choice organizations.—

(A) Enrollment.—Such process shall permit an individual who wishes to elect a Medicare + Choice plan offered by a Medicare + Choice organization to make such election through the filing of an appropriate election form with the organization.

(B) Disenrollment.—Such process shall permit an individual, who has elected a Medicare + Choice plan offered by a Medicare + Choice organization and who wishes to terminate such election, to terminate such election through the filing of an appropriate election form with the organization.

(3) Default.—

(A) Initial election.—

(i) In general.—Subject to clause (ii), an individual who fails to make an election during an initial election period under subsection (e)(1) is deemed to have chosen the original medicare fee-for-service program option.

(ii) Seamless continuation of coverage.—The Secretary may establish procedures under which an individual who is enrolled in a health plan (other than Medicare+Choice plan) offered by a Medicare + Choice organization at the time of the initial election period and who fails to elect to receive coverage other than through the organization is deemed to have elected the Medicare + Choice plan offered by the organization (or, if the organization offers more than one such plan, such plan or plans as the Secretary identifies under such procedures).

(B) Continuing periods.—An individual who has made (or is deemed to have made) an election under this section is considered to have continued to make such election until such time as—

(i) the individual changes the election under this section, or

(ii) the Medicare + Choice plan with respect to which such election is in effect is discontinued or, subject to subsection (b)(1)(B), no longer serves the area in which the individual resides.

(d) Providing Information to Promote Informed Choice.—

(1) In general.—The Secretary shall provide for activities under this subsection to broadly disseminate information to medicare beneficiaries (and prospective medicare beneficiaries) on the coverage options provided under this section in order to promote an active, informed selection among such options.

(2) Provision of notice.—

(A) Open season notification.—At least 15 days before the beginning of each annual, coordinated election period (as defined in subsection (e)(3)(B)), the Secretary shall mail to each Medicare + Choice eligible individual residing in an area the following:

(i) General information.—The general information described in paragraph (3).

(ii) List of plans and comparison of plan options.—A list identifying the Medicare + Choice plans that are (or will be) available to residents of the area and information described in paragraph (4) concerning such plans. Such information shall be presented in a comparative form.

(iii) Additional information.—Any other information that the Secretary determines will assist the individual in making the election under this section. The mailing of such information shall be coordinated, to the extent practicable, with the mailing of any annual notice under section 1804.

(B) Notification to newly eligible medicare + choice eligible individuals.—To the extent practicable, the Secretary shall, not later than 30 days before the beginning of the initial Medicare + Choice enrollment period for an individual described in subsection (e)(1), mail to the individual the information described in subparagraph (A).

(C) Form.—The information disseminated under this paragraph shall be written and formatted using language that is easily understandable by medicare beneficiaries.

(D) Periodic updating.—The information described in subparagraph (A) shall be updated on at least an annual basis to reflect changes in the availability of Medicare + Choice plans and the benefits and Medicare + Choice monthly basic and supplemental beneficiary premiums for such plans.

(3) General information.—General information under this paragraph, with respect to coverage under this part during a year, shall include the following:

(A) Benefits under original medicare fee-for-service program option.— A general description of the benefits covered under the original medicare fee-for-service program under parts A and B, including—

(i) covered items and services,

(ii) beneficiary cost sharing, such as deductibles, coinsurance, and copayment amounts, and (iii) any beneficiary liability for balance billing.

(B) Election procedures.—Information and instructions on how to exercise election options under this section.

(C) Rights.—A general description of procedural rights (including grievance and appeals procedures) of beneficiaries under the original medicare fee-for-service program and the Medicare + Choice program and the right to be protected against discrimination based on health status–related factors under section 1852(b).

(D) Information on medigap and medicare select.—A general description of the benefits, enrollment rights, and other requirements applicable to medicare supplemental policies under section 1882 and provisions relating to medicare select policies described in section 1882(t).

(E) Potential for contract termination.—The fact that a Medicare + Choice organization may terminate its contract, refuse to renew its contract, or reduce the service area included in its contract, under this part, and the effect of such a termination, nonrenewal, or service area reduction may have on individuals enrolled with the Medicare + Choice plan under this part.

(F) Catastrophic Coverage And Single Deductible.—In the case of an MA regional plan, a description of the catastrophic coverage and single deductible applicable under the plan.

(4) Information comparing plan options.—Information under this paragraph, with respect to a Medicare + Choice plan for a year, shall include the following:

(A) Benefits.—The benefits covered under the plan, including the following:

(i) Covered items and services beyond those provided under the original medicare fee-for-service program.

(ii) Any beneficiary cost sharing, including information on the single deductible (if applicable) under section 1858(b)(1).

       (iii) Any maximum limitations on out-of-pocket expenses.

       (iv) In the case of an MSA plan, differences in cost sharing, premiums, and balance billing under such a plan compared to under other Medicare + Choice plans.

       (v) In the case of a Medicare + Choice private fee-for-service plan, differences in cost sharing, premiums, and balance billing under such a plan compared to under other Medicare + Choice plans.

       (vi) The extent to which an enrollee may obtain benefits through out-of-network health care providers.

       (vii) The extent to which an enrollee may select among in- network providers and the types of providers participating in the plan's network.

       (viii) The organization's coverage of emergency and urgently needed care.

   (B) Premiums.—

       (i) In general.—The[315] monthly amount of the premium charged to an individual.[316]

       (ii) Reductions.—The reduction in part B premiums, if any.[317]

The monthly amount of the premium charged to an individual.

   (C) Service area.—The service area of the plan.

   (D) Quality and performance.—To the extent available, plan quality and performance indicators for the benefits under the plan (and how they compare to such indicators under the original medicare fee-for-service program under parts A and B in the area involved), including—

       (i) disenrollment rates for medicare enrollees electing to receive benefits through the plan for the previous 2 years (excluding disenrollment due to death or moving outside the plan's service area),

       (ii) information on medicare enrollee satisfaction,

       (iii) information on health outcomes, and

       (iv) the recent record regarding compliance of the plan with requirements of this part (as determined by the Secretary).

   (E) Supplemental benefits.—Supplemental health care benefits, including any reductions in cost-sharing under section 1852(a)(3) and the terms and conditions (including premiums) for such benefits.

  (5) Maintaining a toll-free number and internet site.—The Secretary shall maintain a toll-free number for inquiries regarding Medicare + Choice options and the operation of this part in all areas in which Medicare + Choice plans are offered and an Internet site through which individuals may electronically obtain information on such options and Medicare + Choice plans.

  (6) Use of non–federal entities.—The Secretary may enter into contracts with non-Federal entities to carry out activities under this subsection.

  (7) Provision of information.—A Medicare + Choice organization shall provide the Secretary with such information on the organization and

each Medicare + Choice plan it offers as may be required for the preparation of the information referred to in paragraph (2)(A).

(e) Coverage Election Periods.—

(1) Initial choice upon eligibility to make election if medicare + choice plans available to individual.—If, at the time an individual first becomes entitled to benefits under part A and enrolled under part B, there is one or more Medicare + Choice plans offered in the area in which the individual resides, the individual shall make the election under this section during a period specified by the Secretary such that if the individual elects a Medicare + Choice plan during the period, coverage under the plan becomes effective as of the first date on which the individual may receive such coverage.

(2) Open enrollment and disenrollment opportunities.—Subject to paragraph (5)—

(A) Continuous open enrollment and disenrollment through 2005.—At any time during the period beginning January 1, 1998, and ending on December 31, 2005, a Medicare + Choice eligible individual may change the election under subsection (a)(1).

(B) Continuous open enrollment and disenrollment for first 6 months during 2006.—

(i) In general.—Subject to clause (ii), at any time during the first 6 months of 2006, or, if the individual first becomes a Medicare + Choice eligible individual during 2006, during the first 6 months during 2006 in which the individual is a Medicare + Choice eligible individual, a Medicare + Choice eligible individual may change the election under subsection (a)(1).

(ii) Limitation of one change.—An individual may exercise the right under clause (i) only once. The limitation under this clause shall not apply to changes in elections effected during an annual, coordinated election period under paragraph (3) or during a special enrollment period under the first sentence of paragraph (4).

(C) Continuous open enrollment and disenrollment for first 3 months in subsequent years.—

(i) In general.—Subject to clause (ii), at any time during the first 3 months of a year after 2006, or, if the individual first becomes a Medicare + Choice eligible individual during a year after 2006, during the first 3 months of such year in which the individual is a Medicare + Choice eligible individual, a Medicare + Choice eligible individual may change the election under subsection (a)(1).

(ii) Limitation of one change during open enrollment period each year.—An individual may exercise the right under clause (i) only once during the applicable 3-month period described in such clause in each year. The limitation under this clause shall not apply to changes in elections effected during an annual, coordinated election period under paragraph (3) or during a special enrollment period under paragraph (4).

(D) Continuous open enrollment for institutionalized individuals.—At any time after 2005 in the case of a Medicare + Choice eligible individual who is institutionalized (as defined by the Secretary), the individual may elect under subsection (a)(1)—

(i) to enroll in a Medicare + Choice plan; or

(ii) to change the Medicare + Choice plan in which the individual is enrolled.

(E) Limited Continuous Open Enrollment of Original Fee-for-Service Enrollees in Medicare Advantage Non-Prescription Drug Plans.—

(i) In general.—On any date during the period beginning on January 1, 2007, and ending on July 31, 2007, [318] on which a Medicare Advantage eligible individual is an unenrolled fee-for-service individual (as defined in clause (ii)), the individual may elect under subsection (a)(1) to enroll in a Medicare Advantage plan that is not an MA-PD plan.

(ii) Unenrolled fee-for-service individual defined.—In this subparagraph, the term "unenrolled fee-for-service individual" means, with respect to a date, a Medicare Advantage eligible individual who—

(I) is receiving benefits under this title through enrollment in the original medicare fee-for-service program under parts A and B;

(II) is not enrolled in an MA plan on such date; and

(III) as of such date is not otherwise eligible to elect to enroll in an MA plan.

(iii) Limitation of one change during the applicable period[319].—An individual may exercise the right under clause (i) only once during the period described in such clause[320].

(iv) No effect on coverage under a prescription drug plan.—Nothing in this subparagraph shall be construed as permitting an individual exercising the right under clause (i)—

(I) who is enrolled in a prescription drug plan under part D, to disenroll from such plan or to enroll in a different prescription drug plan; or

(II) who is not enrolled in a prescription drug plan, to enroll in such a plan.

(3) Annual, coordinated election period.—

(A) In general.—Subject to paragraph (5), each individual who is eligible to make an election under this section may change such election during an annual, coordinated election period.

(B) Annual, coordinated election period.—For purposes of this section, the term 'annual, coordinated election period' means—

(i) with respect to a year before 2002, the month of November before such year;

(ii) with respect to 2002, 2003, 2004, and 2005, the period beginning on November 15 and ending on December 31 of the year before such year;

(iii) with respect to 2006, the period beginning on November 15, 2005, and ending on May 15, 2006; and

(iv) with respect to 2007 and succeeding years, the period beginning on November 15 and ending on December 31 of the year before such year.

(C) Medicare + choice health information fairs.—During the fall season of each year (beginning with 1999), in conjunction with the annual coordinated election period defined in subparagraph (B), the Secretary shall provide for a nationally coordinated educational and publicity campaign to inform Medicare + Choice eligible individuals about Medicare + Choice plans and the election process provided under this section.

(D) Special information campaign in 1998.—During November 1998 the Secretary shall provide for an educational and publicity campaign to inform Medicare + Choice eligible individuals about the availability of Medicare + Choice plans, and eligible organizations with risk-sharing contracts under section 1876, offered in different areas and the election process provided under this section.

(4) Special election periods.—Effective as of January 1, 2006, an individual may discontinue an election of a Medicare + Choice plan offered by a Medicare + Choice organization other than during an annual, coordinated election period and make a new election under this section if—

(A)(i) the certification of the organization or plan under this part has been terminated, or the organization or plan has notified the individual of an impending termination of such certification; or

(ii) the organization has terminated or otherwise discontinued providing the plan in the area in which the individual resides, or has notified the individual of an impending termination or discontinuation of such plan;

(B) the individual is no longer eligible to elect the plan because of a change in the individual's place of residence or other change in circumstances (specified by the Secretary, but not including termination of the individual's enrollment on the basis described in clause (i) or (ii) of subsection (g)(3)(B));

(C) the individual demonstrates (in accordance with guidelines established by the Secretary) that—

(i) the organization offering the plan substantially violated a material provision of the organization's contract under this part in relation to the individual (including the failure to provide an enrollee on a timely basis medically necessary care for which benefits are available under the plan or the failure to provide such covered care in accordance with applicable quality standards); or

(ii) the organization (or an agent or other entity acting on the organization's behalf) materially misrepresented the plan's provisions in marketing the plan to the individual; or

(D) the individual meets such other exceptional conditions as the Secretary may provide.

Effective as of January 1, 2006, an individual who, upon first becoming eligible for benefits under part A at age 65, enrolls in a Medicare + Choice plan under this part, the individual may discontinue the election of such plan, and elect coverage under the original fee-for-service plan, at any time during the 12-month period beginning on the effective date of such enrollment.

    (5) Special rules for msa plans.—Notwithstanding the preceding provisions of this subsection, an individual—

        (A) may elect an MSA plan only during—

           (i) an initial open enrollment period described in paragraph (1), or

           (ii) an annual, coordinated election period described in paragraph (3)(B);

        (B) subject to subparagraph (C), may not discontinue an election of an MSA plan except during the periods described in clause (ii) or (iii) of subparagraph (A) and under the first sentence of paragraph (4); and

        (C) who elects an MSA plan during an annual, coordinated election period, and who never previously had elected such a plan, may revoke such election, in a manner determined by the Secretary, by not later than December 15 following the date of the election.

    (6) Open enrollment periods.—Subject to paragraph (5), a Medicare + Choice organization—

        (A) shall accept elections or changes to elections during the initial enrollment periods described in paragraph (1), during the month of November 1998 and during the annual, coordinated election period under paragraph (3) for each subsequent year, and during special election periods described in the first sentence of paragraph (4); and

        (B) may accept other changes to elections at such other times as the organization provides.

(f) Effectiveness of Elections and Changes of Elections.—

    (1) During initial coverage election period.—An election of coverage made during the initial coverage election period under subsection (e)(1) shall take effect upon the date the individual becomes entitled to benefits under part A and enrolled under part B, except as the Secretary may provide (consistent with section 1838) in order to prevent retroactive coverage.

    (2) During continuous open enrollment periods.—An election or change of coverage made under subsection (e)(2) shall take effect with the first day of the first calendar month following the date on which the election or change is made.

    (3) Annual, coordinated election period.—An election or change of coverage made during an annual, coordinated election period (as defined in subsection (e)(3)(B)) in a year shall take effect as of the first day of the following year.

    (4) Other periods.—An election or change of coverage made during any other period under subsection (e)(4) shall take effect in such manner as the Secretary provides in a manner consistent (to the extent practicable) with protecting continuity of health benefit coverage.

(g) Guaranteed Issue and Renewal.—

(1) In general.—Except as provided in this subsection, a Medicare + Choice organization shall provide that at any time during which elections are accepted under this section with respect to a Medicare + Choice plan offered by the organization, the organization will accept without restrictions individuals who are eligible to make such election.

(2) Priority.—If the Secretary determines that a Medicare + Choice organization, in relation to a Medicare + Choice plan it offers, has a capacity limit and the number of Medicare + Choice eligible individuals who elect the plan under this section exceeds the capacity limit, the organization may limit the election of individuals of the plan under this section but only if priority in election is provided—

(A) first to such individuals as have elected the plan at the time of the determination, and

(B) then to other such individuals in such a manner that does not discriminate, on a basis described in section 1852(b), among the individuals (who seek to elect the plan).

The preceding sentence shall not apply if it would result in the enrollment of enrollees substantially nonrepresentative, as determined in accordance with regulations of the Secretary, of the medicare population in the service area of the plan.

(3) Limitation on termination of election.—

(A) In general.—Subject to subparagraph (B), a Medicare + Choice organization may not for any reason terminate the election of any individual under this section for a Medicare + Choice plan it offers.

(B) Basis for termination of election.—A Medicare + Choice organization may terminate an individual's election under this section with respect to a Medicare + Choice plan it offers if—

(i) any Medicare + Choice monthly basic and supplemental beneficiary premiums required with respect to such plan are not paid on a timely basis (consistent with standards under section 1856 that provide for a grace period for late payment of such premiums),

(ii) the individual has engaged in disruptive behavior (as specified in such standards), or

(iii) the plan is terminated with respect to all individuals under this part in the area in which the individual resides.

(C) Consequence of termination.—

(i) Terminations for cause.—Any individual whose election is terminated under clause (i) or (ii) of subparagraph (B) is deemed to have elected the original medicare fee-for-service program option described in subsection (a)(1)(A).

(ii) Termination based on plan termination or service area reduction.—Any individual whose election is terminated under subparagraph (B)(iii) shall have a special election period under subsection (e)(4)(A) in which to change coverage to coverage under another Medicare + Choice plan. Such an individual who fails to make an election during such period is deemed to have chosen to change coverage to the original medicare fee-for-service program option described in subsection (a)(1)(A).

(D) Organization obligation with respect to election forms.—Pursuant to a contract under section 1857, each Medicare + Choice organization receiving an election form under subsection (c)(2) shall transmit to the Secretary (at such time and in such manner as the Secretary may specify) a copy of such form or such other information respecting the election as the Secretary may specify.

(h) Approval of Marketing Material and Application Forms.—

(1) Submission.—No marketing material or application form may be distributed by a Medicare + Choice organization to (or for the use of) Medicare + Choice eligible individuals unless—

(A) at least 45 days (or 10 days in the case described in paragraph (5)) before the date of distribution the organization has submitted the material or form to the Secretary for review, and

(B) the Secretary has not disapproved the distribution of such material or form.

(2) Review.—The standards established under section 1856 shall include guidelines for the review of any material or form submitted and under such guidelines the Secretary shall disapprove (or later require the correction of) such material or form if the material or form is materially inaccurate or misleading or otherwise makes a material misrepresentation.

(3) Deemed approval (1-stop shopping).—In the case of material or form that is submitted under paragraph (1)(A) to the Secretary or a regional office of the Department of Health and Human Services and the Secretary or the office has not disapproved the distribution of marketing material or form under paragraph (1)(B) with respect to a Medicare + Choice plan in an area, the Secretary is deemed not to have disapproved such distribution in all other areas covered by the plan and organization except with regard to that portion of such material or form that is specific only to an area involved.

(4) Prohibition of certain marketing practices.—Each Medicare + Choice organization shall conform to fair marketing standards, in relation to Medicare + Choice plans offered under this part, included in the standards established under section 1856. Such standards—

(A) shall not permit a Medicare + Choice organization to provide for, subject to subsection (j)(2)(C), cash, gifts, prizes, or other monetary rebates[321] as an inducement for enrollment or otherwise;[322]

(B) may include a prohibition against a Medicare + Choice organization (or agent of such an organization) completing any portion of any election form used to carry out elections under this section on behalf of any individual[323];

(C)[324] shall not permit a Medicare Advantage organization (or the agents, brokers, and other third parties representing such organization) to conduct the prohibited activities described in subsection (j)(1); and

(D)[325] shall only permit a Medicare Advantage organization (and the agents, brokers, and other third parties representing such organization) to conduct the activities described in subsection (j)(2) in accordance with the limitations established under such subsection.

(5) Special treatment of marketing material following model marketing language.—In the case of marketing material of an organization that uses, without modification, proposed model language specified by the Secretary, the period specified in paragraph (1)(A) shall be reduced from 45 days to 10 days.

(6)[326] Required inclusion of plan type in plan name.—For plan years beginning on or after January 1, 2010, a Medicare Advantage organization must ensure that the name of each Medicare Advantage plan offered by the Medicare Advantage organization includes the plan type of the plan (using standard terminology developed by the Secretary).

(7)[327]Strengthening the Ability of States to Act in Collaboration With the Secretary to Address Fraudulent or Inappropriate Marketing Practices.—

  (A) Appointment of agents and brokers.—Each Medicare Advantage organization shall—

    (i) only use agents and brokers who have been licensed under State law to sell Medicare Advantage plans offered by the Medicare Advantage organization;

    (ii) in the case where a State has a State appointment law, abide by such law; and

    (iii) report to the applicable State the termination of any such agent or broker, including the reasons for such termination (as required under applicable State law).

  (B) Compliance with state information requests.—Each Medicare Advantage organization shall comply in a timely manner with any request by a State for information regarding the performance of a licensed agent, broker, or other third party representing the Medicare Advantage organization as part of an investigation by the State into the conduct of the agent, broker, or other third party.

    (i) Effect of Election of Medicare + Choice Plan Option.—

(1) Payments to organizations.—Subject to sections 1852(a)(5), 1853(a) (4), 1853(g), 1853(h), 1886(d)(11), and 1886(h)(3)(D), payments under a contract with a Medicare + Choice organization under section 1853 (a) with respect to an individual electing a Medicare + Choice plan offered by the organization shall be instead of the amounts which (in the absence of the contract) would otherwise be payable under parts A and B for items and services furnished to the individual.

(2) Only organization entitled to payment.—Subject to sections 1853(a)(4), 1853(e), 1853(g), 1853(h), 1857(f)(2), 1858(h), 1886(d)(11), and 1886 (h)(3)(D), only the Medicare + Choice organization shall be entitled to receive payments from the Secretary under this title for services furnished to the individual.

(j)[328]Prohibited Activities Described and Limitations on the Conduct of Certain Other Activities.—

(1) Prohibited activities described—The following prohibited activities are described in this paragraph:

    (A) Unsolicited means of direct contact.—Any unsolicited means of direct contact of prospective enrollees, including soliciting door-to-door or any outbound telemarketing without the prospective enrollee initiating contact.

    (B) Cross-selling.—The sale of other non-health related products (such as annuities and life insurance) during any sales or marketing activity or presentation conducted with respect to a Medicare Advantage plan.

    (C) Meals.—The provision of meals of any sort, regardless of value, to prospective enrollees at promotional and sales activities.

    (D) Sales and marketing in health care settings and at educational events.—Sales and marketing activities for the enrollment of individuals in Medicare Advantage plans that are conducted—

        (i) in health care settings in areas where health care is delivered to individuals (such as physician offices and pharmacies), except in the case where such activities are conducted in common areas in health care settings; and

        (ii) at educational events.

(2)[329] Limitations.—The Secretary shall establish limitations with respect to at least the following:

    (A) Scope of marketing appointments.—The scope of any appointment with respect to the marketing of a Medicare Advantage plan. Such limitation shall require advance agreement with a prospective enrollee on the scope of the marketing appointment and documentation of such agreement by the Medicare Advantage organization. In the case where the marketing appointment is in person, such documentation shall be in writing.

    (B) Co-branding.—The use of the name or logo of a co-branded network provider on Medicare Advantage plan membership and marketing materials.

    (C) Limitation of gifts to nominal dollar value.—The offering of gifts and other promotional items other than those that are of nominal value (as determined by the Secretary) to prospective enrollees at promotional activities

    (D) Compensation.—The use of compensation other than as provided under guidelines established by the Secretary. Such guidelines shall ensure that the use of compensation creates incentives for agents and brokers to enroll individuals in the Medicare Advantage plan that is intended to best meet their health care needs.

    (E) Required training, annual retraining, and testing of agents, brokers, and other third parties.—The use by a Medicare Advantage organization of any individual as an agent, broker, or other third party representing the organization that has not completed an initial training and testing program and does not complete an annual retraining and testing program.

PART D—VOLUNTARY PRESCRIPTION DRUG BENEFIT PROGRAM[416]

Subpart 1—Part D Eligible Individuals and Prescription Drug Benefits

Eligibility, Enrollment, and Information

Sec. 1860D-1. [42 U.S.C. 1395w-101]

(a) Provision of Qualified Prescription Drug Coverage Through Enrollment In Plans.—

(1) In general.—Subject to the succeeding provisions of this part, each part D eligible individual (as defined in paragraph (3)(A)) is entitled to obtain qualified prescription drug coverage (described in section 1860D-2(a)) as follows:

(A) Fee-for-service enrollees may receive coverage through a prescription drug plan.—A part D eligible individual who is not enrolled in an MA plan may obtain qualified prescription drug coverage through enrollment in a prescription drug plan (as defined in section 1860D-41(a)(14)).

(B) Medicare advantage enrollees.—

(i) Enrollees in a plan providing qualified prescription drug coverage receive coverage through the plan.—A part D eligible individual who is enrolled in an MA-PD plan obtains such coverage through such plan.

(ii) Limitation on enrollment of MA plan enrollees in prescription drug plans.—Except as provided in clauses (iii) and (iv), a part D eligible individual who is enrolled in an MA plan may not enroll in a prescription drug plan under this part.

(iii) Private fee-for-service enrollees in MA plans not providing qualified prescription drug coverage permitted to enroll in a prescription drug plan.—A part D eligible individual who is enrolled in an MA private fee-for-service plan (as defined in section 1859 (b)(2)) that does not provide qualified prescription drug coverage may obtain qualified prescription drug coverage through enrollment in a prescription drug plan.

(iv) Enrollees in MSA plans permitted to enroll in a prescription drug plan.—A part D eligible individual who is enrolled in an MSA plan (as defined in section 1859(b)(3)) may obtain qualified prescription drug coverage through enrollment in a prescription drug plan.

(2) Coverage first effective January 1, 2006.—Coverage under prescription drug plans and MA-PD plans shall first be effective on January 1, 2006.

(3) Definitions.—For purposes of this part:

(A) Part D eligible individual.—The term "part D eligible individual" means an individual who is entitled to benefits under part A or enrolled under part B.

(B) MA plan.—The term "MA plan" has the meaning given such term in section 1859(b)(1).

(C) MA-PD plan.—The term "MA-PD plan" means an MA plan that provides qualified prescription drug coverage.

(b) Enrollment Process For Prescription Drug Plans.—

(1) Establishment of process.—

(A) In general.—The Secretary shall establish a process for the enrollment, disenrollment, termination, and change of enrollment of part D eligible individuals in prescription drug plans consistent with this subsection.

(B) Application of MA rules.—In establishing such process, the Secretary shall use rules similar to (and coordinated with) the rules for enrollment, disenrollment, termination, and change of enrollment with an MA-PD plan under the following provisions of section 1851:

(i) Residence requirements.—Section 1851(b)(1)(A), relating to residence requirements.

(ii) Exercise of choice.—Section 1851(c) (other than paragraph (3) (A) of such section), relating to exercise of choice.

(iii) Coverage election periods.—Subject to paragraphs (2) and (3) of this subsection, section 1851(e) (other than subparagraphs (B), (C) and (E) of paragraph (2) and the second sentence of paragraph (4) of such section), relating to coverage election periods, including initial periods, annual coordinated election periods, special election periods, and election periods for exceptional circumstances.

(iv) Coverage periods.—Section 1851(f), relating to effectiveness of elections and changes of elections.

(v) Guaranteed issue and renewal.—Section 1851(g) (other than paragraph (2) of such section and clause (i) and the second sentence of clause (ii) of paragraph (3)(C) of such section), relating to guaranteed issue and renewal.

(vi) Marketing material and application forms.—Section 1851(h), relating to approval of marketing material and application forms. In applying clauses (ii), (iv), and (v) of this subparagraph, any reference to section 1851(e) shall be treated as a reference to such section as applied pursuant to clause (iii) of this subparagraph.

(C) Special rule.—The process established under subparagraph (A) shall include, in the case of a part D eligible individual who is a full-benefit dual eligible individual (as defined in section 1935(c)(6)) who has failed to enroll in a prescription drug plan or an MA-PD plan, for the enrollment in a prescription drug plan that has a monthly beneficiary premium that does not exceed the premium assistance available under section 1860D-14(a)(1)(A)). If there is more than one such plan available, the Secretary shall enroll such an individual on a random basis among all such plans in the PDP region. Nothing in the previous sentence shall prevent such an individual from declining or changing such enrollment.

(2) Initial enrollment period.—

(A) Program initiation.—In the case of an individual who is a part D eligible individual as of November 15, 2005, there shall be an initial enrollment period that shall be the same as the annual, coordinated open election period described in section 1851(e)(3)(B)(iii), as applied under paragraph (1)(B)(iii).

(B) Continuing periods.—In the case of an individual who becomes a part D eligible individual after November 15, 2005, there shall be an initial enrollment period which is the period under section 1851(e)(1), as applied under paragraph (1)(B)(iii) of this section, as if "entitled to benefits under part A or enrolled under part B" were substituted for "entitled to benefits under part A and enrolled under part B," but in no case shall such period end before the period described in subparagraph (A).

(3) Additional special enrollment periods.—The Secretary shall establish special enrollment periods, including the following:

(A) Involuntary loss of creditable prescription drug coverage.—

   (i) In general.—In the case of a part D eligible individual who involuntarily loses creditable prescription drug coverage (as defined in section 1860D-13(b)(4)).

   (ii) Notice.—In establishing special enrollment periods under clause (i), the Secretary shall take into account when the part D eligible individuals are provided notice of the loss of creditable prescription drug coverage.

   (iii) Failure to pay premium.—For purposes of clause (i), a loss of coverage shall be treated as voluntary if the coverage is terminated because of failure to pay a required beneficiary premium.

   (iv) Reduction in coverage.—For purposes of clause (i), a reduction in coverage so that the coverage no longer meets the requirements under section 1860D-13(b)(5) (relating to actuarial equivalence) shall be treated as an involuntary loss of coverage.

(B) Errors in enrollment.—In the case described in section 1837(h) (relating to errors in enrollment), in the same manner as such section applies to part B.

(C) Exceptional circumstances.—In the case of part D eligible individuals who meet such exceptional conditions (in addition to those conditions applied under paragraph (1)(B)(iii)) as the Secretary may provide.

(D) Medicaid coverage.—In the case of an individual (as determined by the Secretary) who is a full-benefit dual eligible individual (as defined in section 1935(c)(6)).

(E) Discontinuance of MA-PD election during first year of eligibility.— In the case of a part D eligible individual who discontinues enrollment in an MA-PD plan under the second sentence of section 1851 (e)(4) at the time of the election of coverage under such sentence under the original medicare fee-for-service program.

(4) Information to facilitate enrollment.—

(A) In general.—Notwithstanding any other provision of law but subject to subparagraph (B), the Secretary may provide to each PDP sponsor and MA organization such identifying information about part D eligible individuals as the Secretary determines to be necessary to facilitate efficient marketing of prescription drug plans and MA-PD plans to such individuals and enrollment of such individuals in such plans.

(B) Limitation.—

(i) Provision of information.—The Secretary may provide the information under subparagraph (A) only to the extent necessary to carry out such subparagraph.

(ii) Use of information.—Such information provided by the Secretary to a PDP sponsor or an MA organization may be used by such sponsor or organization only to facilitate marketing of, and enrollment of part D eligible individuals in, prescription drug plans and MA-PD plans.

(5) Reference to enrollment procedures for MA-PD plans.—For rules applicable to enrollment, disenrollment, termination, and change of enrollment of part D eligible individuals in MA-PD plans, see section 1851.

(6) Reference to penalties for late enrollment.—Section 1860D-13(b) imposes a late enrollment penalty for part D eligible individuals who—

(A) enroll in a prescription drug plan or an MA-PD plan after the initial enrollment period described in paragraph (2); and

(B) fail to maintain continuous creditable prescription drug coverage during the period of non-enrollment.

(c) Providing information to beneficiaries.—

(1) Activities.—The Secretary shall conduct activities that are designed to broadly disseminate information to part D eligible individuals (and prospective part D eligible individuals) regarding the coverage provided under this part. Such activities shall ensure that such information is first made available at least 30 days prior to the initial enrollment period described in subsection (b)(2)(A).

(2) Requirements.—The activities described in paragraph (1) shall—

(A) be similar to the activities performed by the Secretary under section 1851(d), including dissemination (including through the toll-free telephone number 1-800-MEDICARE) of comparative information for prescription drug plans and MA-PD plans; and

(B) be coordinated with the activities performed by the Secretary under such section and under section 1804.

(3) Comparative information.—

(A) In general.—Subject to subparagraph (B), the comparative information referred to in paragraph (2)(A) shall include a comparison of the following with respect to qualified prescription drug coverage:

(i) Benefits.—The benefits provided under the plan.

(ii) Monthly beneficiary premium.—The monthly beneficiary premium under the plan.

(iii) Quality and performance.—The quality and performance under the plan.

(iv) Beneficiary cost-sharing.—The cost-sharing required of part D eligible individuals under the plan.

(v) Consumer satisfaction surveys.—The results of consumer satis-faction surveys regarding the plan conducted pursuant to section 1860D-4(d).
(B) Exception for unavailability of information.—The Secretary is not required to provide comparative information under clauses (iii) and (v) of subparagraph (A) with respect to a plan—
(i) for the first plan year in which it is offered; and
(ii) for the next plan year if it is impracticable or the information is otherwise unavailable.
(4) Information on late enrollment penalty.—The information dissemi-nated under paragraph (1) shall include information concerning the methodology for determining the late enrollment penalty under section 1860D-13(b).

Prescription Drug Benefits

Sec. 1860D-2. [42 U.S.C. 1395w-102]

(a) Requirements.—
(1) In general.—For purposes of this part and part C, the term "qualified prescription drug coverage" means either of the following:
(A) Standard prescription drug coverage with access to negotiated prices.—Standard prescription drug coverage (as defined in subsec-tion (b)) and access to negotiated prices under subsection (d).
(B) Alternative prescription drug coverage with at least actuarially equivalent benefits and access to negotiated prices.—Coverage of covered part D drugs which meets the alternative prescription drug coverage requirements of subsection (c) and access to negoti-ated prices under subsection (d), but only if the benefit design of such coverage is approved by the Secretary, as provided under subsection (c).
(2) Permitting supplemental prescription drug coverage.—
(A) In general.—Subject to subparagraph (B), qualified prescription drug coverage may include supplemental prescription drug coverage consisting of either or both of the following:
(i) Certain reductions in cost-sharing.—
(I) In general.—A reduction in the annual deductible, a reduction in the coinsurance percentage, or an increase in the initial cov-erage limit with respect to covered part D drugs, or any combi-nation thereof, insofar as such a reduction or increase increases the actuarial value of benefits above the actuarial value of basic prescription drug coverage.
(II) Construction.—Nothing in this paragraph shall be construed as affecting the application of subsection (c)(3).
(ii) Optional drugs.—Coverage of any product that would be a covered part D drug but for the application of subsection (e)(2)(A).
(B) Requirement.—A PDP sponsor may not offer a prescription drug plan that provides supplemental prescription drug coverage pursuant

to subparagraph (A) in an area unless the sponsor also offers a prescription drug plan in the area that only provides basic prescription drug coverage.

(3) Basic prescription drug coverage.—For purposes of this part and part C, the term "basic prescription drug coverage" means either of the following:

(A) Coverage that meets the requirements of paragraph (1)(A).

(B) Coverage that meets the requirements of paragraph (1)(B) but does not have any supplemental prescription drug coverage described in paragraph (2)(A).

(4) Application of secondary payor provisions.—The provisions of section 1852(a)(4) shall apply under this part in the same manner as they apply under part C.

(5) Construction.—Nothing in this subsection shall be construed as changing the computation of incurred costs under subsection (b)(4).

(b) Standard Prescription Drug Coverage.—For purposes of this part and part C, the term "standard prescription drug coverage" means coverage of covered part D drugs that meets the following requirements:

(1) Deductible.—

(A) In general.—The coverage has an annual deductible—

(i) for 2006, that is equal to $250; or

(ii) for a subsequent year, that is equal to the amount specified under this paragraph for the previous year increased by the percentage specified in paragraph (6) for the year involved.

(B) Rounding.—Any amount determined under subparagraph (A)(ii) that is not a multiple of $5 shall be rounded to the nearest multiple of $5.

(2) Benefit structure.—

(A) 25 percent coinsurance.—The coverage has coinsurance (for costs above the annual deductible specified in paragraph (1) and up to the initial coverage limit under paragraph (3)) that is—

(i) equal to 25 percent; or

(ii) actuarially equivalent (using processes and methods established under section 1860D-11(c)) to an average expected payment of 25 percent of such costs.

(B) Use of tiers.—Nothing in this part shall be construed as preventing a PDP sponsor or an MA organization from applying tiered copayments under a plan, so long as such tiered copayments are consistent with subparagraph (A)(ii).

(3) Initial coverage limit.—

(A) In general.—Except as provided in paragraph (4), the coverage has an initial coverage limit on the maximum costs that may be recognized for payment purposes (including the annual deductible)—

(i) for 2006, that is equal to $2,250; or

(ii) for a subsequent year, that is equal to the amount specified in this paragraph for the previous year, increased by the annual percentage increase described in paragraph (6) for the year involved.

(B) Rounding.—Any amount determined under subparagraph (A)(ii) that is not a multiple of $10 shall be rounded to the nearest multiple of $10.

(4) Protection against high out-of-pocket expenditures.—

    (A) In general.—

        (i) In general.—The coverage provides benefits, after the part D eligible individual has incurred costs (as described in subparagraph (C)) for covered part D drugs in a year equal to the annual out-of-pocket threshold specified in subparagraph (B), with cost-sharing that is equal to the greater of—

            (I) a copayment of $2 for a generic drug or a preferred drug that is a multiple source drug (as defined in section 1927(k)(7)(A)(i)) and $5 for any other drug; or

            (II) coinsurance that is equal to 5 percent.

        (ii) Adjustment of amount.—For a year after 2006, the dollar amounts specified in clause (i)(I) shall be equal to the dollar amounts specified in this subparagraph for the previous year, increased by the annual percentage increase described in paragraph (6) for the year involved. Any amount established under this clause that is not a multiple of a 5 cents shall be rounded to the nearest multiple of 5 cents.

    (B) Annual out-of-pocket threshold.—

        (i) In general.—For purposes of this part, the "annual out-of-pocket threshold" specified in this subparagraph—

            (I) for 2006, is equal to $3,600; or

            (II) for a subsequent year, is equal to the amount specified in this subparagraph for the previous year, increased by the annual percentage increase described in paragraph (6) for the year involved.

        (ii) Rounding.—Any amount determined under clause (i)(II) that is not a multiple of $50 shall be rounded to the nearest multiple of $50.

    (C) Application.—In applying subparagraph (A)—

        (i) incurred costs shall only include costs incurred with respect to covered part D drugs for the annual deductible described in paragraph (1), for cost-sharing described in paragraph (2), and for amounts for which benefits are not provided because of the application of the initial coverage limit described in paragraph (3), but does not include any costs incurred for covered part D drugs which are not included (or treated as being included) in the plan's formulary; and

        (ii) such costs shall be treated as incurred only if they are paid by the part D eligible individual (or by another person, such as a family member, on behalf of the individual), under section 1860D-14, or under a State Pharmaceutical Assistance Program and the part D eligible individual (or other person) is not reimbursed through insurance or otherwise, a group health plan, or other third-party payment arrangement (other than under such section or such a Program) for such costs.

(D) Information regarding third-party reimbursement.—
  (i) Procedures for exchanging information.—In order to accurately apply the requirements of subparagraph (C)(ii), the Secretary is authorized to establish procedures, in coordination with the Secretary of the Treasury and the Secretary of Labor—
    (I) for determining whether costs for part D eligible individuals are being reimbursed through insurance or otherwise, a group health plan, or other third-party payment arrangement; and
    (II) for alerting the PDP sponsors and MA organizations that offer the prescription drug plans and MA-PD plans in which such individuals are enrolled about such reimbursement arrangements.
  (ii) Authority to request information from enrollees.—A PDP sponsor or an MA organization may periodically ask part D eligible individuals enrolled in a prescription drug plan or an MA-PD plan offered by the sponsor or organization whether such individuals have or expect to receive such third-party reimbursement. A material misrepresentation of the information described in the preceding sentence by an individual (as defined in standards set by the Secretary and determined through a process established by the Secretary) shall constitute grounds for termination of enrollment in any plan under section 1851(g)(3)(B) (and as applied under this part under section 1860D-1(b)(1)(B)(v)) for a period specified by the Secretary.

(5) Construction.—Nothing in this part shall be construed as preventing a PDP sponsor or an MA organization offering an MA-PD plan from reducing to 0 the cost-sharing otherwise applicable to preferred or generic drugs.

(6) Annual percentage increase.—The annual percentage increase specified in this paragraph for a year is equal to the annual percentage increase in average per capita aggregate expenditures for covered part D drugs in the United States for part D eligible individuals, as determined by the Secretary for the 12-month period ending in July of the previous year using such methods as the Secretary shall specify.

(c) Alternative Prescription Drug Coverage Requirements.—A prescription drug plan or an MA-PD plan may provide a different prescription drug benefit design from standard prescription drug coverage so long as the Secretary determines (consistent with section 1860D-11(c)) that the following requirements are met and the plan applies for, and receives, the approval of the Secretary for such benefit design:

(1) Assuring at least actuarially equivalent coverage.—
  (A) Assuring equivalent value of total coverage.—The actuarial value of the total coverage is at least equal to the actuarial value of standard prescription drug coverage.
  (B) Assuring equivalent unsubsidized value of coverage.—The unsubsidized value of the coverage is at least equal to the unsubsidized value of standard prescription drug coverage. For purposes of this

subparagraph, the unsubsidized value of coverage is the amount by which the actuarial value of the coverage exceeds the actuarial value of the subsidy payments under section 1860D-15 with respect to such coverage.

(C) Assuring standard payment for costs at initial coverage limit.—The coverage is designed, based upon an actuarially representative pattern of utilization, to provide for the payment, with respect to costs incurred that are equal to the initial coverage limit under subsection (b)(3) for the year, of an amount equal to at least the product of—

(i) the amount by which the initial coverage limit described in subsection (b)(3) for the year exceeds the deductible described in subsection (b)(1) for the year; and

(ii) 100 percent minus the coinsurance percentage specified in subsection (b)(2)(A)(i).

(2) Maximum required deductible.—The deductible under the coverage shall not exceed the deductible amount specified under subsection (b)(1) for the year.

(3) Same protection against high out-of-pocket expenditures.—The coverage provides the coverage required under subsection (b)(4).

(d) Access to Negotiated Prices.—

(1) Access.—

(A) In general.—Under qualified prescription drug coverage offered by a PDP sponsor offering a prescription drug plan or an MA organization offering an MA-PD plan, the sponsor or organization shall provide enrollees with access to negotiated prices used for payment for covered part D drugs, regardless of the fact that no benefits may be payable under the coverage with respect to such drugs because of the application of a deductible or other cost-sharing or an initial coverage limit (described in subsection (b)(3)).

(B) Negotiated prices.—For purposes of this part, negotiated prices shall take into account negotiated price concessions, such as discounts, direct or indirect subsidies, rebates, and direct or indirect remunerations, for covered part D drugs, and include any dispensing fees for such drugs.

(C) Medicaid-related provisions.—The prices negotiated by a prescription drug plan, by an MA-PD plan with respect to covered part D drugs, or by a qualified retiree prescription drug plan (as defined in section 1860D-22(a)(2)) with respect to such drugs on behalf of part D eligible individuals, shall (notwithstanding any other provision of law) not be taken into account for the purposes of establishing the best price under section 1927(c)(1)(C).

(2) Disclosure.—A PDP sponsor offering a prescription drug plan or an MA organization offering an MA-PD plan shall disclose to the Secretary (in a manner specified by the Secretary) the aggregate negotiated price concessions described in paragraph (1)(B) made available to the sponsor or organization by a manufacturer which are passed through in the form of lower subsidies, lower monthly beneficiary prescription drug

premiums, and lower prices through pharmacies and other dispensers. The provisions of section 1927(b)(3)(D) apply to information disclosed to the Secretary under this paragraph.

(3) Audits.—To protect against fraud and abuse and to ensure proper disclosures and accounting under this part and in accordance with section 1857(d)(2)(B) (as applied under section 1860D-12(b)(3)(C)), the Secretary may conduct periodic audits, directly or through contracts, of the financial statements and records of PDP sponsors with respect to prescription drug plans and MA organizations with respect to MA-PD plans.

(e) Covered Part D Drug Defined.—

(1) In general.—Except as provided in this subsection, for purposes of this part, the term "covered part D drug" means—

(A) a drug that may be dispensed only upon a prescription and that is described in subparagraph (A)(i), (A)(ii), or (A)(iii) of section 1927 (k)(2); or

(B) a biological product described in clauses (i) through (iii) of subparagraph (B) of such section or insulin described in subparagraph (C) of such section and medical supplies associated with the injection of insulin (as defined in regulations of the Secretary),

and such term includes a vaccine licensed under section 351 of the Public Health Service Act[417] (and, for vaccinations administered on or after January 1, 2008, its administration) and any use of a covered part D drug for a medically accepted indication (as defined in paragraph (4))[418].

(2) Exclusions.—

(A) In general.—Such term does not include drugs or classes of drugs, or their medical uses, which may be excluded from coverage or otherwise restricted under section 1927(d)(2), other than subparagraph (E) of such section (relating to smoking cessation agents),[419] or under section 1927(d)(3), as such sections were in effect on the date of the enactment of this part. Such term also does not include a drug when used for the treatment of sexual or erectile dysfunction, unless such drug were used to treat a condition, other than sexual or erectile dysfunction, for which the drug has been approved by the Food and Drug Administration.

(B) Medicare covered drugs.—A drug prescribed for a part D eligible individual that would otherwise be a covered part D drug under this part shall not be so considered if payment for such drug as so prescribed and dispensed or administered with respect to that individual is available (or would be available but for the application of a deductible) under part A or B for that individual.

(3) Application of general exclusion provisions.—A prescription drug plan or an MA-PD plan may exclude from qualified prescription drug coverage any covered part D drug—

(A) for which payment would not be made if section 1862(a) applied to this part; or

(B) which is not prescribed in accordance with the plan or this part. Such exclusions are determinations subject to reconsideration and appeal pursuant to subsections (g) and (h), respectively, of section 1860D-4.

(4)[420] Medically accepted indication defined.—

    (A) In general.—For purposes of paragraph (1), the term "medically accepted indication" has the meaning given that term—

        (i) in the case of a covered part D drug used in an anticancer chemotherapeutic regimen, in section 1861(t)(2)(B), except that in applying such section—

            (I) "prescription drug plan or MA-PD plan" shall be substituted for "carrier" each place it appears; and

            (II) subject to subparagraph (B), the compendia described in section 1927(g)(1)(B)(i)(III) shall be included in the list of compendia described in clause (ii)(I) section 1861(t)(2)(B); and

        (ii) in the case of any other covered part D drug, in section 1927(k)(6).

    (B) Conflict of interest.—On and after January 1, 2010, subparagraph (A)(i)(II) shall not apply unless the compendia described in section 1927(g)(1)(B)(i)(III) meets the requirement in the third sentence of section 1861(t)(2)(B).

    (C) Update.—For purposes of applying subparagraph (A)(ii), the Secretary shall revise the list of compendia described in section 1927(g)(1)(B)(i) as is appropriate for identifying medically accepted indications for drugs. Any such revision shall be done in a manner consistent with the process for revising compendia under section 1861(t)(2)(B).

Notes

[3] See Vol. II, P.L. 101-239, §6011(b), with respect to determining the payment amount for services to hemophilia inpatients.

[4] See Vol. II, P.L. 108-173, §923(d)(2), with respect to a study and report on the accuracy and consistency of information provided through the toll-free telephone number 1-800-MEDICARE.

[5] See Vol. II, P.L. 104-191, §203(b).

[10] See Vol. II, P.L. 108-173, §925, with respect to the inclusion of additional information in notices to beneficiaries about skilled nursing facility benefits.

[12] P.L. 110-275, §185, added §1809, effective July 15, 2008.

[13] See Vol. II, P.L. 101-508, §4004, with respect to payments for medical education costs.

See Vol. II, P.L. 110-275, §169, with respect to a MEDPAC study and report on Medicare Advantage payments.

[18] P.L. 108-271, §8(b), provided that "Any reference to the General Accounting Office in any law, rule, regulation, certificate, directive, instruction, or other official paper in force on the date of enactment of this Act (July 7, 2004) shall be considered to refer and apply to the Government Accountability Office."

[19] As in original.

[20] See §1886(d)(5)(F)(iv).

[21] See Vol. II, Code of Federal Regulations, Title 42.

[22] See Vol. II, P.L. 108-173, §405(c)(2), with respect to the development of alternative timing methods of periodic interim payments.

[23] See Vol. II, P.L. 101-508, §4005(c)(3), with respect to guidance for intermediaries and hospitals.

[24] P.L. 108-173, §911(b)(3); 117 Stat. 2383.

[25] P.L. 108-173, §911(b)(4)(A); 117 Stat. 2383.

[26] See Vol. II, 31 U.S.C. 3902(a).

[27] P.L. 108-173, §911(b)(5); 117 Stat. 2383.

[28] See Vol. II, P.L. 108-173, §801, with respect to inclusion in annual report of Medicare Trustees of information on status of Medicare Trust Funds.

[29] See Vol. II, P.L. 83-591, §3101(b) and 3111(b).

[30] P.L. 83-591.

P.L. 99-514, §2, provides, except when inappropriate, any reference to the Internal Revenue Code of 1954 shall include a reference to the Internal Revenue Code of 1986.

[31] See Vol. II, P.L. 83-591, §1401(b).

[32] See Vol. II, P.L. 108-173, §801(a).

See Vol. II, P.L. 108-203, §413, with respect to the reinstatement of certain reporting requirements.

[33] See Vol. II, 31 U.S.C. 3111.

[34] See Vol. II, P.L. 83-591, §3101(b).

[35] P.L. 83-591.

[36] See Vol. II, P.L. 104-191, §242(b), with respect to criminal fines deposited in Federal Hospital Insurance Trust Fund and§249(c), with respect to property forfeited deposited in Federal Hospital Insurance Trust Fund.

[37] See Vol. II, P.L. 83-591, §9601.

[38] See Vol. II, 18 U.S.C. 24(a).

[39] October 30, 1972 [P.L. 92-603; 86 Stat. 1374].

[40] See Vol. II, P.L. 89-97.

[57] See Vol. II, P.L. 98-369, §2323(e), with respect to monitoring of hepatitis vaccine.

See Vol. II, P.L. 101-239, §6112(b), with respect to rental payments for enteral and parenteral pumps; and §6113(c) and (e), with respect to the development of criteria regarding consultation with a physician.

See Vol. II, P.L. 103-66, §13515(b), with respect to budget neutrality adjustment.

See Vol. II, P.L. 109-171, §5107(b), with respect to with respect to the implementation of clinically appropriate code edits in order to identify and eliminate improper payments for therapy services.

See Vol. II, P.L. 110-275, §169, with respect to a MEDPAC study and report on Medicare Advantage payments.

[58] P.L. 110-275, §143(b)(1)(A), struck out "and outpatient" and substituted, "outpatient."

[59] P.L. 110-275, §143(b)(1)(B), inserted, "and outpatient speech-language pathology services (other than services to which the second sentence of section 1861(p) applies through the application of section 1861(ll)(2))," **to be applicable to services furnished on or after July 1, 2009**. See Vol. II, P.L. 110-275, §143(d), with respect to a rule of construction regarding existing regulations and policies.

[60] See Vol. II, P.L. 108-173, §416, with respect to treatment of certain clinical diagnostic laboratory tests furnished to hospital outpatients in certain rural areas and §733, with respect to payments for pancreatic islet cell investigational transplants for medicare beneficiaries in clinical trials.

[145] P.L. 110-275, §143(b)(4)(A), strikes out "1861(g)" and substitutes "subsection (g) or (ll)(2) of section 1861," **applicable to services furnished on or after July 1, 2009.**

[146] P.L. 110-275, §143(b)(4)(A), strikes out "1861(g)" and substitutes "subsection (g) or (ll)(2) of section 1861," **applicable to services furnished on or after July 1, 2009.**

[147] P.L. 110-275, §143(b)(4)(B), inserts "or outpatient speech-language pathology services, respectively," **applicable to services furnished on or after July 1, 2009.**

[148] P.L. 110-275, §143(b)(4)(A), strikes out "1861(g)" and substitutes "subsection (g) or (ll)(2) of section 1861," **applicable to services furnished on or after July 1, 2009.**

[153] See Vol. II, P.L. 75-162.

[154] See Vol. II, P.L. 83-591, §7701(a)(38).

[190] P.L. 75-162 [as amended by P.L. 93-445].

[227] See Vol. II, P.L. 106-554, §1(a)(6)[542], with respect to treatment of certain physician pathology services under Medicare.

See Vol. II, P.L. 108-173, §303(a)(2), with respect to the treatment of other services currently in non-physician work pool, and §303(a)(3), with respect to payment for multiple chemotherapy agents furnished on a single day through the push technique; §303(a)(5), with respect to MEDPAC review and reports and secretarial response.

See Vol. II, P.L. 109-432, §101(e), with respect to the transfer of funds for implementation of the amendments made by P.L. 109-432, Division B, Title I, §101(a), (b) and (d), which added §1848(d)(7), (k) and (l), respectively.

See Vol. II, P.L. 110-275, §131(b)(4)(B), with respect to billing for audiology services, and §138, with respect to an adjustment for Medicare mental health services.

[314] See Vol. II, P.L. 108-173, §231(e), with respect to a study on the impact of specialized MA plans for special needs individuals.

See Vol. II, P.L. 110-173, §108(b), with respect to a moratorium on the designation of plans and the enrollment in new plans.

See Vol. II, P.L. 110-275, §168, with respect to a MEDPAC study and report on quality measures.

[315] P.L. 106-554, §606((c)(i), struck out "Premiums.—" and substituted "Premiums.—"

(i) In General.—The," applicable to years beginning with 2003.

[316] P.L. 108-173, §222(l)(3)(B)(iii), struck out "Medicare + Choice monthly basic beneficiary premium and Medicare + Choice monthly supplemental beneficiary premium, if any, for the plan or, in the case of an MSA plan, the Medicare + Choice monthly MSA premium" and substituted "the monthly amount of the premium charged to an individual," applicable to plan years beginning on or after January 1, 2006.

[317] P.L. 106-554, §606((c)(ii), added clause (ii), applicable to years beginning with 2003.

[318] P.L. 110-48, §2(1), struck out "2007 or 2008" and substituted "the period beginning on January 1, 2007, and ending on July 31, 2007," effective July 18, 2007.

[319] P.L. 110-48, §2(2)(A), struck out "year" and substituted "the applicable period," effective July 18, 2007.

[320] P.L. 110-48, §2(2)(A), struck out "the year" and substituted "the period described in such clause," effective July 18, 2007.

[321] P.L. 110-275, §103(a)(1)(A)(i)(I)(aa), struck out "cash or monetary rebates" and substituted, "subject to subsection (j)(2)(C), cash, gifts, prizes, or other monetary rebates," applicable to plan years beginning on or after January 1, 2009.

[322] P.L. 110-275, §103(a)(1)(A)(i)(I)(bb), struck out, "and" and inserted a semicolon.

[323] P.L. 110-275, §103(a)(1)(A)(i)(II), struck out the period and inserted a semicolon.

[324] P.L. 110-275, §103(a)(1)(A)(i)(III), added subparagraph (C), applicable to plan years beginning on or after January 1, 2009.

[325] P.L. 110-275, §103(b)(1)(A), added subparagraph (D), to take effect on a date specified by the Secretary (but in no case later than November 15, 2008).

[326] P.L. 110-275, §103(c)(1), added paragraph (6), effective July 15, 2008.

[327] P.L. 110-275, §103(d)(1), added paragraph (7), applicable to plan years beginning on or after January 1, 2009.

[328] P.L. 110-275, §103(a)(1)(A)(ii), added subsection (j), applicable to plan years beginning on or after January 1, 2009.

[329] P.L. 110-275, §103(b)(1)(B), added paragraph (2), to take effect on a date specified by the Secretary (but in no case later than November 15, 2008).

[416] See Vol. II, P.L. 108-173, §101(b), with respect to the submission of a legislative proposal; §101(c), with respect to a study on transitioning Part B prescription drug coverage; §101(d), with respect to a report on progress in implementation of prescription drug benefit; §106, with respect to the State Pharmaceutical Assistance Transition commission; and §110, with respect to a conflict of interest study.

[417] See Vol. II, P.L. 78-410, §351.

[418] P.L. 110-275, §182(a)(1), struck out "(as defined in section 1927(k)(6))" and substituted "(as defined in paragraph (4))," effective January 1, 2009.

[419] P.L. 110-275, §175(a), inserts other than subparagraph (I) of such section (relating to barbiturates) if the barbiturate is used in the treatment of epilepsy, cancer, or a chronic mental health disorder, and other than subparagraph (J) of such section (relating to benzodiazepines)," **to be applicable to prescriptions dispensed on or after January 1, 2013**.

[420] P.L. 110-275, §182(a)(1)(B), added paragraph (4), applicable to plan years beginning on or after January 1, 2009.

Appendix B

Timeline for Enactment and Major Changes in Medicare[1]

This timeline details Medicare milestones and highlights major legislative changes. Also included are milestones with related programs such as Medicaid, SCHIP, and where appropriate, Social Security.

1935	On August 13th, President Roosevelt signed the Social Security legislation, creating a new social insurance program in the United States. This legislation formed a work-related, contributory system in which workers would provide for their own pensions as they aged through their contributions to the system. Certain key features, such as disability insurance and health insurance, although discussed in the early planning for the program, were not included.
1945	President Truman requests that Congress establish a national health insurance plan.
	Two decades of debate follow with opponents warning about dangers from "socialized medicine."
1960	Congress passed the Kerr-Mills Act which authorized distribution of federal funds to the states to provide medical assistance to the aged. These funds were provided on a 50 to 80 percent matching basis, with higher percentages going to poorer states. This legislation is seen as a forerunner to the Medicaid legislation, Title XIX of the Social Security legislation. It was enacted in place of a Medicare-type program providing health insurance benefits to elderly Social Security recipients.
1965 **January**	President Johnson's first legislative message to the 89th Congress, *Advancing the Nation's Health*, details a

program that includes hospital insurance for the aged via Social Security and health care for needy children.

March–July   By substantial vote majorities, the House of Representatives (307–116) and the Senate (70–24) passed the "Mills Bill" (H.R. 6675), a package of health benefits and Social Security improvements.

July 30   As part of his "Great Society," President Johnson signs into law (H.R. 6675) to establish Medicare for the elderly and its companion program, Medicaid to insure indigent recipients. Medicare is Title XVIII of the Social Security Act and Medicaid is Title XIX of the Social Security Act. Medicare is a federal program that provides coverage for all people 65 and over under Part A; people must choose Part B. Medicaid expands upon the goals of and replaces the Kerr-Mills Act of 1960. It is a federal-state partnership program in which voluntarily participating states receive grants for those eligible in a state to access a defined set of medical and long-term care benefits.

Former President Truman is the first Medicare enrollee.

Medicare Part A deductible: $40/year.

Medicare Part B premium: $3/month.

1966
July 1   Medicare coverage began. Medicare covered all persons age 65 and over automatically under Part A. Coverage also began for people who signed up for the voluntary medical insurance program (Part B). Over 19 million people 65 and older were enrolled in Medicare at the beginning of the program.

1972
October 30   President Nixon signs the Social Security Amendments of 1972 (PL 92-603) which is the first major adjustment to Medicare. The Bill extends Medicare eligibility to people under age 65 with long-term disabilities (who were receiving SSDI payments for two years) and to individuals with end-stage renal disease (ESRD). The Amendments also make changes beyond eligibility, by establishing professional standards review organizations (PSROs) to review patient care, encouraging the use of health maintenance organizations (HMOs), and giving Medicare the authority to conduct demonstration programs.

Medicare benefits were expanded to include some chiropractic services, speech therapy, and physical therapy.

1973   Coverage for people receiving Social Security Disability Insurance (SSDI) cash payments for two or more years actually begins, along with the ESRD program. Almost two million people under age 65 with long-term disabilities or ESRD are covered.

1977 The Department of Health, Education and Welfare, (DHEW), under Secretary Joseph Califano, creates the Health Care Financing Administration (HCFA) as the agency to administer both the Medicare and Medicaid programs. Before this, the program was administered through Social Security Administration.

1980 A number of changes to Medicare are passed as part of the Omnibus Reconciliation Act of 1980. Changes include expanded home health services by eliminating the limit on the number of home health visits, the prior hospitalization requirement, and the deductible for any Part B benefits. This Act begins an exploration of surgical procedures that could be done on an outpatient basis in an ambulatory surgical center and would be reimbursed on a prospective payment system. The "Baucus Amendments" provide oversight and coordination to Medicare supplemental insurance, also called "Medigap," and establishes a voluntary certification program for Medigap policies.

1981 The Omnibus Budget Reconciliation Act of 1981 (OBRA 1981) includes provisions to slow growth in Medicare spending. As part of this Act, inpatient hospital deductible is increased.

1982 The Tax Equity and Fiscal Responsibility Act (TEFRA) increases the Part B premium to cover 25 percent of program costs. This is the part of policies, as with those enacted in 1981, designed to slow the growth of Medicare spending. TEFRA facilitates HMOs' participation in the Medicare program and establishes a risk-based prospective payment system for these plans. The Act also expands HCFA's quality oversight efforts by replacing Professional Standards Review Organizations (PSROs) with Peer Review Organizations (PROs). TEFRA imposes a ceiling on the amount Medicare will pay for a hospital discharge. Planning for the future, HHS is required to submit a plan for prospective payments to hospitals and nursing homes. TEFRA requires federal employees to begin paying the HI payroll tax. As an expansion of services, hospice services for the terminally ill are added. The Medicare Hospice Benefit in 1982 spurred the rapid growth of hospice programs across the United States. To qualify for hospice care, patients were required to have a life expectancy of six months or less, as determined by their attending physician, and sign a form which acknowledged their terminal condition and waived their traditional Medicare coverage (which paid for curative medical care) in favor of the palliative (non-curative) care offered by hospice. The Medicare Benefit reimbursed hospices by means of a standard per diem rate of payment per patient, which was presumed to cover the costs of all goods and services provided to patients.

1983   A major overhaul in payment of hospitals is established, with Social Security amendments of 1983 putting in place an inpatient hospital prospective payment system (PPS) for Medicare. The PPS is based on diagnosis-related groups, or DRGs, a pre-determined payment for treating a specific condition. This system replaces cost-based payments. Because of TEFRA requirement that federal employees pay into Medicare, most federal civilian employees become covered by Medicare.

1984   Remaining federal employees, including the President, members of Congress, and the federal judiciary are covered.

As part of continuing efforts to hold down rising costs, growth in Medicare spending, and the federal deficit, the Deficit Reduction Act of 1984 (DEFRA) freezes physician fees, establishes the Participating Physicians' Program, and establishes fee schedules for laboratory services.

1985   The Consolidated Omnibus Budget Reconciliation Act of 1985 (COBRA) makes Medicare coverage mandatory for newly hired state and local employees, following the precedent of previous years to add federal employees to the system. COBRA establishes the Emergency Medical Treatment and Labor Act (EMTALA), which requires hospitals that participate in Medicare and operate active ERs provide appropriate medical screenings and stabilizing treatments.

The Emergency Extension Act of 1985 freezes PPS payment rates for inpatient hospital care and continues the physician payment freeze, as part of a continued effort to slow the growth of Medicare spending.

1986   Medicare expands services by making hospice benefits for the terminally ill permanent. Omnibus Budget Reconciliation Act of 1986 (OBRA 1986) revises payment procedures for various Medicare services in order to help slow the growth in Medicare spending.

1987   The Omnibus Budget Reconciliation Act of 1987 (OBRA 1987) modifies payments to providers as part of a continuing effort to lower costs and deal with the deficit. In the quality area, this legislation imposes quality standards for Medicare- and Medicaid-certified nursing homes, to deal with well-documented quality problems facing individuals in nursing homes. The Balanced Budget and Emergency Deficit Control Reaffirmation Act of 1987 freezes Medicare payment rates, as part of another effort to slow Medicare spending.

The Medicare and Medicaid Patient and Program Protection Act of 1987 focuses upon improving antifraud efforts and strengthening beneficiary protection programs.

1988   The Medicare Catastrophic Coverage Act of 1988 is the largest expansion of the program since its enactment. This major overhaul of Medicare benefits is enacted with a particular focus on providing coverage for catastrophic illness and prescription drugs. It includes an outpatient prescription drug benefit and expanded hospital and skilled nursing facility benefits. For those Medicare recipients who also receive Medicaid, Medicare premiums and cost-sharing are reimbursed by the Medicaid program. In the quality area, the Clinical Laboratory Improvement Amendments are enacted to improve quality performance requirements for clinical laboratories in an effort to provide more accurate and reliable laboratory tests. To move toward catastrophic coverage, a bipartisan Commission on Comprehensive Health Care (which became known as "Pepper Commission" after the late Congressman Claude Pepper of Florida) is established to address the feasibility of a long-term care benefit under Medicare.

1989   As a reaction to the negative public response to aspects of the 1988 legislation, the Medicare Catastrophic Coverage Repeal Act of 1989 retracts major provisions of the 1988 Medicare Catastrophic Coverage Act before the legislation really becomes operational. This includes both removal of outpatient drug benefit and the out-of-pocket limit. Quality aspects of the Bill remain in force, as does the "Pepper Commission."

The Omnibus Budget Reconciliation Act of 1989 (OBRA 1989) establishes the Resource-Based Relative Value Scale (RBRVS) for physicians, replacing charge-based payments. Limits are placed upon physician balance billing. In addition, physicians are prohibited from referring Medicare patients to clinical laboratories in which they have a financial interest. This legislation also contains a number of other provisions designed to slow the growth in Medicare spending.

1990

The Omnibus Budget Reconciliation Act of 1990 (OBRA 1990) establishes the Specified Low-Income Medicare Beneficiary (SLMB) eligibility group. This requires state Medicaid programs to cover premiums for beneficiaries with incomes between 100 and 120 percent of the federal poverty level. Service expansions include coverage of screening mammography and partial hospitalization services in community mental health centers. Federal standards are established for Medigap policies, including standardized benefit packages and minimum loss ratios, replacing the voluntary certification system.

Despite the recommendations of the U.S. Bipartisan Commission on Comprehensive Health Care (the "Pepper Commission") for the creation of a new Medicare long-term care program to provide nursing home and home- and community-based services, this does not occur.

1993

The Omnibus Budget Reconciliation Act of 1993 modifies payments to Medicare providers, again as part of an overall push for deficit reduction. In addition, to help protect the fiscal solvency of Medicare funds, the cap on wages subject to the HI payroll tax is lifted.

1996

The Health Insurance Portability and Accountability Act of 1996 (HIPAA) establishes the Medicare Integrity Program, which provides funds for program integrity activities.

The Personal Responsibility and Work Opportunity Act of 1996 (PRWOA) repeals the AFDC individual entitlement to cash assistance and replaced it with the Temporary Assistance for Needy Families (TANF) block grant to states. This ends the formal linkage between cash assistance (welfare) and Medicaid eligibility, a major shift in Medicaid.

1997

The Balanced Budget Act of 1997 (BBA) includes a wide range of changes in provider payments to slow the growth in Medicare spending as part of the legislation to balance the federal budget. The Medicare + Choice program, a new structure for Medicare HMOs and other private health plans, is offered to beneficiaries. Some service expansion continues to occur. The BBA requires HCFA to develop and implement five new Medicare prospective payment systems: inpatient rehabilitation hospital or unit services; skilled nursing facility services; home health services; hospital outpatient services; and outpatient rehabilitation services. The Law also provides additional assistance with Medicare Part B premiums for beneficiaries with incomes between 120 and 135 percent of poverty (QI-1s) through a first-come, first-serve block grant program administered by state Medicaid programs. The Law provided for partial assistance with premiums for beneficiaries with incomes between 135 and 175 percent of poverty (QI-2s). The BBA also establishes the National Advisory Commission on the Future of Medicare and the Medicare Payment Advisory Commission (which replace earlier groups such as the Prospective Payment Assessment Commission and the Physician Payment Review Commission).

The Balanced Budget Act of 1997 (BBA 97) also establishes the State Children's Health Insurance Program (SCHIP), one of the largest expansions in provision of health insurance to selected groups of U.S. children since the initial passage of Medicaid in 1965. This program allows states to cover uninsured children in families with incomes below 200 percent of FPL and who are ineligible for Medicaid. The federal funds are capped, but the matching rate for costs of SCHIP services is enhanced (30 percent higher than a state's Medicaid matching rate), with a federal match of 65 percent as a floor and 85 percent as a ceiling.

1998   As a way to improve the access of the general public to information about Medicare, the Internet site www.Medicare.gov is launched to provide updated information.

1999   Continuing with the focus on providing the public with better services at lower cost, a toll-free number, 1-800-MEDICARE (1-800-633-4227), is made available nationwide as an additional way to disseminate information to those interested in Medicare. The first annual *Medicare & You* handbook was mailed to all Medicare beneficiary households.

The Ticket to Work and Work Incentives Improvements Act of 1999 (TWWIIA) expands the availability of Medicare and Medicaid for certain disabled beneficiaries who return to work.

Adjustments to payment schedules and fees occurs when the Balanced Budget Refinement Act of 1999

(BBRA) increases payments for some Medicare providers and reduces or freezes payment rates for other Medicare services. Payments to Medicare + Choice plans are also increased.

The National Advisory Commission on the Future of Medicare completes its report on Medicare reform, but there are not enough Congressional votes to make a formal recommendation.

2000

The Medicare, Medicaid, and SCHIP Benefits Improvement and Protection Act (BIPA) of 2000 continues to modify payments to providers, and in this case, increases Medicare payments to providers and Medicare + Choice plans. This legislation created payment floors for urban areas and increased the payment floor for rural areas, reduced certain Medicare beneficiary copayments, and added coverage for preventive services. BIPA also enabled people with amyotrophic lateral sclerosis (ALS or Lou Gehrig's disease) to enroll in Medicare upon diagnosis, instead of having to satisfy the 24-month waiting period.

2001

The Centers for Medicare and Medicaid Services (CMS) becomes the name for the agency administering Medicare and Medicaid, replacing the Health Care Financing Administration. Coverage for people with ALS actually begins.

2002

The Public Health Security and Bioterrorism Preparedness and Response Act of 2002, includes a number of public health measures, but also temporarily moves deadlines for submitting Medicare + Choice plan information. The law states that in 2005, individuals enrolled in Medicare + Choice plans may only make and change elections to these plans on a limited basis. This is later changed by the Medicare Modernization Act of 2003.

2003

The Consolidated Appropriations Resolution (CAR) of 2003 increases payments for some hospitals, updates the physician fee schedule, and makes changes in premium payments for some Part B recipients.

December 8

The Medicare Prescription Drug, Improvement, and Modernization Act of 2003 (MMA) is passed by the House (220–215) and the Senate (54–44) in November and signed into law (Public Law 108-173) by President George W. Bush. This provides a new outpatient prescription drug benefit under Medicare beginning in 2006. In the interim, it creates a temporary prescription drug discount card and transitional assistance program. In addition to the major drug benefit aspect of this bill, the MMA also establishes a new income-related Part B premium for beneficiaries with higher incomes (beginning in 2007), indexes the Part B deductible, creates regional PPOs under the Medicare Advantage program (previously named Medicare + Choice), along with special needs plans, and also includes financial and other incentives for private health plans to contract with Medicare. The MMA begins changes in the ways of assessing Medicare's financial status by reviewing general revenues as a share of total Medicare spending.

2004   A temporary Medicare-Approved Drug Discount Card Program begins. This is a transitional program, as is another transitional program to provide a $600 annual credit to low-income Medicare beneficiaries without prescription drug coverage in 2004 and 2005.

2005   Medicare begins covering a "Welcome to Medicare" physical, along with other preventive services, such as cardiovascular screening blood tests and diabetes screening tests. Medicare also begins education and outreach activities to implement the 2006 prescription drug benefit.

November 15, 2005–
May 15, 2006   These are the dates for the first open enrollment period for Medicare Prescription Drug Plan (PDP) or a Medicare Advantage Prescription Drug Plan (MAPD).

2006   In January 2006, the Medicare Drug Benefit begins. Medicare beneficiaries begin receiving subsidized prescription drug coverage through Part D plans. As required by law, the Medicare Trustees calculate for the first time that general revenues will exceed 45 percent of total Medicare outlays within a seven-year period.

2007   Medicare beneficiaries with higher incomes (greater than $80,000/individual; $160,000/couple) begin to pay a higher monthly Part B premium. This is based on their modified adjusted gross income, ranging from $105.80 to $161.40 per month.

For the second consecutive year, the Medicare Board of Trustees calculate that general revenue will exceed 45 percent of Medicare funding within the succeeding seven years, triggering a "Medicare funding warning."

In December 2007, the Medicare, Medicaid, and SCHIP Extension Act of 2007 (PL 110-173) is signed into law. The Act prevents a 10.1 percent reduction in Medicare physician payments that had been scheduled for 2008 and gives physicians a 0.5 percent increase through June 30, 2008.

2008   In July 2008, the Medicare Improvements for Patients
and Providers Act of 2008 (MIPPA) is signed into law
(PL 110-275) with many features similar to the Act
passed in 2007. For example, the Bill prevents a reduction in physician fees through the end of 2008, and
increases fees by 1.1 percent through 2009. Because
these changes are supposed to be revenue neutral, the
cost of the postponement of physician fee cuts is offset
by cutting bonus payments to Medicare Advantage
plans. The Act also provides benefit expansions or
improvements by reducing coinsurance for mental
health visits, eliminating the deductible for the "Welcome to Medicare" exam, increasing allowable resources for low-income beneficiaries applying for the
Medicare Savings Programs (MSP) and modifying the
definition of excludable assets in determining Low-
Income Subsidy (LIS) program eligibility. As a response
to the "Medicare funding warning" issued in 2007,
the President submits a proposals to Congress to
reduce the share of general revenues as a share of total
spending, as required by law. Also, as in 2006 and 2007,
the Medicare Trustees issue a "Medicare funding
warning" in 2008, as required by law, indicating general revenues will exceed 45 percent of total Medicare
spending within a seven-year period. The MIPPA also
included changes in payments to Advantage (HMO/
managed care plans), and added beneficiary protections,
focusing on marketing practices for those enrolled in
these plans.

Medicare beneficiaries with incomes exceeding
$82,000/individual and $164,000/couple pay income-
related Part B premiums of up to $238.40.

2009–2010   The U.S. House of Representatives passed the Senate-
passed bill to reform health care in March 2010 by a
vote of 220 to 211. The House also passed a bill which
then was sent back to the Senate to modify versions of
the Senate bill; that bill was passed in March, 2010.
The initial Senate version of the bill was passed in late
2009. The final Bill was signed by President Obama on
March 23, 2010. When fully phased in, the legislation
will cover around 32 million Americans who are currently uninsured. Major coverage expansion begins in
2014, but beginning in 2010, insurers must remove lifetime dollar limits on policies. Medicaid will be
expanded, the "donut hole" in the Medicare drug plan
will gradually disappear, and certain preventive services
in Medicare will be available without a copayment.

There will be reductions in Medicare Advantage plan payments that will help to extend the life of the Medicare Trust Fund. An independent advisory board will be created to help make recommendations for other cost savings. There will be elimination of Part D cost sharing for dual eligible recipients. The legislation will establish the Community First Choice Option, which will create a state plan option under section 1915 of the Social Security Act, to provide community-based attendant support and services to individuals with disabilities who are Medicaid-eligible and require an institutional level of care. It will create demonstration programs for certain types of home care and modifications to some of the rules for nursing homes that receive Medicare payments, related to transparencies of how actions occur.

NOTE

1. Many details related to Medicare and Medicaid are from the Medicare and Medicaid timelines available through the Kaiser Family Foundation Web site (www.KFF.org). More details are available at that source.

Glossary

Access to Care Ability of persons needing health care services to obtain appropriate care in a timely manner. While access to care is not the same as having health insurance coverage, such coverage (either private or public such as Medicare or Medicaid) is a major factor in having access to care.

Agency for Health Care Research and Quality (AHRQ) Agency that deals with issues related to health care policy, health services research, health quality issues, and health practice guidelines. The AHRQ also conducts several important surveys to obtain data on health care expenditures and some hospital-related data. Earlier versions of the agency were Agency for Health Care Policy and Research (AHCPR) and National Center for Health Services Research (NCHSR).

Assisted Living Facilities Living facilities, usually specifically for the aging population, that provide aid. Some provide independent living options where residents maintain their own apartments, yet are offered transportation to shopping and to health care facilities, as well as dining facilities. Some facilities offer smaller personal living places in which there may be a small bedroom, bathroom, and a living room that combines a sitting and eating area with limited kitchen facilities. This model also provides daily supervision of a person's medication. In these settings, people may be transported to three meals a day. In most states, there is not much regulation of these types of long-term care options, as contrasted with nursing home settings, which are reimbursable by Medicare following an illness or by Medicaid. Generally, neither Medicare nor Medicaid pay for assisted living facilities, although some private long-term care policies do reimburse for assisted living facilities.

Capitation A set amount, or a flat rate, that is paid to cover a person's medical care for a specified period of time, often a month or a year.

Center for Medicare and Medicaid Services (CMMS) Formerly known as the Health Care Financing Administration (HCFA), this agency administers the Medicare, Medicaid, and SCHIP programs.

Chronic Disease A persistent medical condition. Chronic problems may lead to permanent health care problems. Examples of chronic diseases include diabetes, heart disease, and chronic obstructive pulmonary disease (COPD). Care for chronic diseases can occur in many settings, such as outpatient, hospitals, or long-term care facilities.

Community First Choice Option Part of the new Obama health reform legislation, passed in March 2010 that will create a state plan option under section 1915 of the Social Security Act. Provides community-based attendant supports and services to individuals with disabilities who are Medicaid-eligible and who require an institutional level of care.

Copayment A portion of the health care expenses that patients must provide. Generally, a health insurance plan, HMO, or Medicare will specify the amount. A copayment is generally paid each time a person receives health care services.

Deductible A portion of health care costs that the insured person must first pay before insurance reimbursement begins. Generally, most plans provide a coverage year, which could coincide with the calendar year, or with some other time period, such as from July through June. A person will pay the costs for health care they receive until the deductible amount is met, and then generally health insurance will begin to cover the costs. Often the copayment will persist. In Medicare, many people buy supplemental insurance to cover deductibles (and copayments) that are part of fee-for-service (FFS) Medicare, that is, traditional Medicare.

Department of Health and Human Services (DHHS) The federal agency that deals with many health-related issues. Agencies such as the National Institutes of Health are part of the DHHS.

Diagnosis-related Group (DRG) The current payment approach used for Medicare hospital payments. Rather than paying for specific services as they occur in the hospital, hospital charges are paid in a bundled group of services as stipulated by a federally specified list of diagnoses. This approach of paying for hospital care has also been incorporated by some private health insurance companies.

Disability Physical or mental handicap that results from injury or illness. These often impact a person's ability to perform important life tasks. For example, a person who is blind has a visual disability and a person who is deaf has a hearing disability. Examples of other types of physical disabilities are the need to use a wheelchair or a prosthetic device for movement of the legs and ambulation, or for movement of the hands in the upper body. As people age, the number of disabilities may increase and many people without disabilities when young and middle-aged develop them when they are older. This is particularly true with sensory disabilities such as loss of vision or hearing.

Entitlement Programs Health care programs to which certain categories of people are entitled. An example is Medicare; most people at age 65 are entitled because of payment of their payroll taxes during years when they were employed.

Fee-for-service (FFS) Payment of specific fees (generally to a physician) for each service that a patient receives, such as an office examination, a shot (immunization), or a diagnostic test. Medicare is generally a FFS system, unless a person is enrolled in Medicare Advantage, the HMO version of Medicare.

Formulary List of acceptable prescription drugs that a health plan or managed care company allows. In many health plans, there may be higher copayments for non-generic formulary drugs than for generic versions of formulary drugs. If a drug is not listed in the formulary of the health insurance plan (including Medicare drug coverage plans), then no payment will be made for that prescription.

Gatekeeper Physician Generally, a primary care physician who functions as the regular source of care for a patient. This provider must approve the use of specialists and other services, most often as part of a managed care plan.

Generalist A family practice, general internal medicine, or general pediatrics physician. These types of physicians often function as gatekeepers within certain managed care systems, including within Medicare.

Gross Domestic Product (GDP) The measure of all the goods and services produced by a nation in a given year.

Health Maintenance Organization (HMO) A type of managed care organization that provides comprehensive medical care for a predetermined annual fee per employee, generally with only modest copayments and small or no deductibles. A trend over the last few years has been increases in the sizes of copayments as ways to keep the basic health insurance costs lower.

Home Health Services Nursing, special therapy services such as physical therapy, and health-related homemaker services that are provided to patients in their home. Services are generally for patients who have a chronic illness or a disability that makes the patient unable to leave their home to receive services.

Hospital Services The health care services patients receive while an overnight patient in a hospital. Analogous to inpatient services.

Hospice Services An array of special services for patients that are dying. Generally these are a blend of medical, spiritual, legal, and family support services and can be delivered in the patient's home, a nursing home, or a special facility designed for this purpose.

Independent Practice Association (IPA) Legal entity with membership comprised of physicians in private practice. The organization can represent physicians in private practice in the negotiation of contracts with managed care organizations.

Inpatient Services Services received while a patient is in a hospital or nursing home, where they stay overnight. Analogous to hospital services.

Insurance Carrier The insurer.

Insured The person who contracts with an insurance company for coverage; also known as the policy holder or the subscriber.

Lifecare Communities Places where, in exchange for a one-time entrance fee plus a monthly maintenance fee, a person receives a guarantee of assisted living, personal care, and nursing home services as needed.

Lifetime Cap Maximum amount of money a health insurance policy will pay over the lifetime of the insured person. Limitations on these caps have become major issues for people who develop serious health problems, and the removal of such limits has been one topic of discussion in recent health care reform approaches. Medicare does not include lifetime caps on most services.

Long-term Care Services received as part of extended care for people with chronic illnesses, mental illnesses, or serious disabilities. These services are often provided in nursing homes, but can also be provided as part of home-based services and often focus on basic daily needs. In recent decades, the provision of care through assisted living facilities has provided some long-term care services outside of a nursing home, but in a special setting.

Managed Care A system of provision and payment for health care that unites the functions of health insurance and the actual delivery of care.

Managed Care Organization (MCO) A term used with similar meanings to Health Maintenance Organization. It is a way of providing care that uses a structure to help a patient organize care from the primary level to more advanced care. In some managed care organizations, there may be specific lists of providers, hospitals, and drugs that may be used. A managed care organization generally provides comprehensive medical care for a predetermined annual fee per employee, typically with only modest copayments and small or no deductibles. A trend in recent years has been increases in the sizes of copayments as ways to keep the basic health insurance costs lower.

Medicaid A joint federal-state program that provides health insurance coverage to many of the poor in the United States. This is a program that is means-tested for which people must provide proof of their income (and in some states, proof of resources such as the value of a home, a car, and money in bank accounts) to qualify for benefits.

Medicare The federal program that provides health insurance coverage to the elderly and some disabled people. Part A covers hospital costs, Part B covers physician and provider costs, and Part D is a newer drug coverage option. The major payer for health insurance for most people over 65 in the United States, although many people also have supplemental health insurance coverage (sometimes called Medigap plans) that pays for health care not covered at all, nor covered completely by Medicare.

Medigap Commercial health insurance policies purchased by people with Medicare coverage to cover the expenses not covered by Medicare; the insurance also provides coverage for certain other costs within Medicare, such as required copayments and deductibles for certain services.

Morbidity Sickness

Mortality Death

National Institutes of Health (NIH) The major research arm of the federal government, as related to health. It includes institutes such as the National Cancer Institute, and its headquarters are located in Bethesda, Maryland. It is the major federal funder of health research, and, in addition, also conducts research.

Nursing Homes Facilities where the most seriously ill elderly (and some non-elderly) with chronic health problems receive long-term care. These types of institutions are subject to federal and state regulation, and generally will have some registered nurses available at all times (in contrast to assisted living facilities), although they are generally not able to provide care for new, acute health care problems as they develop.

Organized Medicine The activities of physicians, generally to protect their own interests, organized through groups such as the American Medical Association.

Outcome Results of health care delivery. Of great interest now as a way to measure the effectiveness of the health care delivery system.

Out-of-pocket Costs Costs of health care that are paid by the patient—the consumer of services; depending upon the type of health insurance, this would include deductibles and copayments for care.

Outpatient Services Health care services that do not require overnight stay in a hospital (as contrasted to inpatient services).

Payer Party that actually makes the payment for services covered by an insurance policy. Generally, the payer is the same as the insurer.

Physician-hospital Organization A legal entity that is formed between a hospital and a physician group, generally to share a market, patients, and other mutual interests.

Preferred Provider Organization (PPO) These types of organizations are related to managed care plans. Often insurance companies set up their own contracts with companies and with providers for the provision of care. In these types of groups, the insurance company makes a contractual arrangement with a group of providers or individual providers for provision of services, typically at a negotiated and discounted fee.

Premiums Amount charged by an insurance company for a policy.

Primary Care Medical care provided in an office or clinic setting by a provider such as a doctor, physician's assistant, or nurse practitioner. Generally, this is the first level of contact by a patient within the health care delivery system and the entry point into health care.

Prospective Payment System (PPS) System in which payment amounts for service is predetermined, as contrasted with retrospective reimbursement. The DRG payment system for hospital care under Medicare is an example of a prospective payment system.

Reimbursement Amount paid to a provider (i.e., doctor, hospital) by the insurance company or managed care group. This payment may only be a portion of what the provider charges. In a managed care setting, the amount is usually negotiated in advance.

Resource-based Relative Value System (RBRVS) The Medicare system used to determine physician fees. Each treatment or visit with a physician is assigned a "relative value" based upon the training, skill, and time that is required to treat the condition.

Retrospective Reimbursement The amount paid for health care service as determined upon the basis of the actual costs incurred, generally after services have been delivered.

Safety Net Programs that enable people to receive health care services (as well as many other social services) when they lack the personal resources to pay for those services. Medicaid is an example of a safety net program in health care, as are community health centers. These are generally government programs.

Single-Payer A proposal for health care reform that emphasizes the creation of a single organization, typically a government agency, to pay all health care claims. While many experts argue this is the best and least expensive way to provide health care access to most of a population, it has not been a popular approach in the recent rounds of discussion of health care reform within the United States. In many ways, traditional FFS Medicare functions as a single-payer system, although the actual job of claims payment is often contracted to private insurance companies but they follow the rules of Medicare set by the federal government.

State Child Health Insurance Program (SCHIP) This program was passed in 1997 as part of the Balanced Budget Act of that year. It was the largest expansion of health coverage since the passage of Medicare and Medicaid. It is a joint federal-state health care program, as is Medicaid. The program focuses on providing coverage for children of the working poor.

Uncompensated Care Services provided to patients as a charity without the patient paying for the services.

Usual, Customary, and Reasonable (UCR) Maximum charges that an insurer will reimburse for a specific service. Typically, each insurance company determines its own UCR, as part of community or statewide surveys of what providers charge.

Welfare Programs Means-tested programs that provides services, whether health or social, to those with low incomes. In health care, Medicaid is an example of a welfare program.

REFERENCE SOURCES

Agency for Healthcare Research and Quality (AHRQ). Coronary angiography is underused for both Medicare managed care and fee-for-service heart attack patients. 2000. http://www.ahrq.gov/research/nov00/1100RA1.htm.

Berenson, Robert A. and Bryan E. Dowd. Medicare advantage Plans at a Crossroads—Yet Again. *Health Affairs* 28(1): w29–w40, 2009. (Published online on November 24, 2008;10.1377/hlthaff.28.2.w29.)

Berkowitz, S. A.; G. Gerstenblith; and G. F. Anderson. Medicare Prescription Drug Coverage Gap. *JAMA* 297(8), 868–870, 2007.

Blevins, Sue. *Medicare's Midlife Crisis*. Washington, D.C.: Cato Institute, 2001.

Blumenthal, David; Moon, Marilyn; Warshawsky, Mark; and Cristina Coccutie (Eds.). *Long-term Care and Medicare Policy: Can We Improve the Continuity of Care?* Washington, D. C.: National Academy of Social Insurance, 2003.

Caffareta, Gail. Private Health Insurance of the Medicare Population and the Baucus Legislation. *Medical Care* 23 (August): 1086–1096, 1985.

Cassel, Christine K. *Medicare Matters: What Geriatric Medicine Can Teach American Health Care*. Berkeley, CA: University of California Press, 2005.

Cassil, Alwyn. 86 Percent of Uninsured Kids in NM Eligible but not Enrolled in Medicaid. *American Medical News*. November 17, p. 4, 1977.

Chapen, Rosemary and Glenn Silloway. Incentive Payments to Nursing Homes Based on Quality of Care. *Journal of Applied Gerontology* 11(2): 131–145, June 1992.

Christensen, Sandra. Medicare + Choice Provisions in the Balanced Budget Act of 1997. *Health Affairs* 17: 224–231, 1998.

Christianson, Jon B. Did 1980s Legislation Slow Medicare Spending? *Health Affairs* 10: 135–142, 1991.

Colamery, S. N. (Ed.) *Medicare: Current Issues and Background*. New York, Nova Science Publishers, Inc., 2003.

Coleman, Barbara. *Trends in Medicaid Long-term Care Spending.* AARP Policy Institute. January, 1999. http://www.aarp.org/research/ppi/ltc/ltc-medicaid/articles/aresearch-import-646-DD38.html.

Cook, Fay Lomax and Edith J. Barrett. *Support for the American Welfare State: The Views of Congress and the Public.* New York: Columbia University Press, 1992.

Corrigan, Janet and Dwight McNeill. Building Organizational Capacity: A Cornerstone of Health Care Reform. *Health Affairs* 28(2): w205–w215, 2009.

Crosson, Francis J. Medicare: The Place to Start Delivery System Reform. *Health Affairs* 28(2): w232–w234, 2009.

Culyer, John and Joseph P. Newhouse (Eds.). *Handbook of Health Economics, Volume 1, Part 2.* Oxford, England: Elsevier Press, 2000.

Davidoff, Amy J.; Garrett, Bowen; Makuc, Diane M.; and Matthew Schirmer. Children Eligible for Medicaid but Not Enrolled: How Great a Policy Concern? *New Federalism: Issues and Options for the State.* Number A–41. Urban Institute, 2000. http://newfederalism.urban.org/html/anf_a41.html.

DesHarnais, Susan; Kobrinski, E.; and John Chesney. The Early Effects of the PPS on Inpatient Utilization and the Quality of Care. *Inquiry* 24: 7–16, 1987.

Edwards, W. O. and C. R. Fisher. Medicare Physician and Hospital Utilization and Expenditure Trends. *Health Care Financing Review* 11: 111–116, 1989.

Epstein, Arnold and David Blumenthal. Physician Payment Reform: Past and Future. *Milbank Quarterly* 71(2): 195–215, 1993.

Executive and Legislative Branches of Both Parties Underfund the Centers for Medicare and Medicaid Services. http://content.healthaffairs.org/cgi/content/abstract/hlthaff.28.4.w688. 2009.

Federal Interagency Forum on Child and Family Statistics. *America's Children: Key National Indicators of Well-Being, 2001.* 2001. www.childstats.gov/ac2001/ac01.asp.

Fisher, Elliot; McClellan, Mark B.; Bertko, John; Lieberman, Steven M.; Lee, Julie J.; Lewis, Julie L.; and Jonathan S. Skinner. Fostering Accountable Health Care: Moving Forward in Medicare. *Health Affairs* 28(2): w219–w231, 2009.

Fisher, Erin and Margie Rosenberg. Medicare Part D: An Evaluation of the Prescription Drug Benefit. Center for Biology Education, pp. 57–63, 2007. http://cbe.wisc.edu/assets/docs/pdf/srp-bio/2007/Fisher.pdf.

Garfinkel, Steven; Bonito, Arthur; and Kenneth McElroy. Socioeconomic Factors and Medicare Supplemental Insurance. *Health Care Financing Review* 9(Fall): 21–30, 1987.

Gay, Greer; Kronenfeld, Jennie J.; Baker, Sam; and Roger Amidon. An Appraisal of Organizational Response to Fiscally Constraining Regulation. *Journal of Health and Social Behavior* 30: 41–55, 1989.

Ginsberg, Paul and Phillip R. Lee. Defending U.S. Physician Payment Reform. *Health Affairs* 8(4): 61–71, 1989.

Glaser, William. The Politics of Paying American Physicians. *Health Affairs* 8(3): 129–146, 1989.

Gold, Marsha. Medicare's Private Plans: A Report Card on Medicare Advantage. *Health Affairs* 28(1): w41–w54, 2009. (Published online November 24, 2008;10.1377/hlthaff.28.1.w41.)

Greene, J.; Blustein, J.; and K. A. Laflamme. Use of preventive care services, beneficiary characteristics, and Medicare HMO performance. *Health Care Financing Review* 22(4), 141–153, 2001.

Guterman, S. and A. Dobson. Impact of the Medicare Prospective Payment System for Hospitals. *Health Care Financing Review* 7: 97–114, 1986.

Hacker, J. How Not to Fix Medicare [Op-Ed]. *The New York Times.* July 2nd, 2003, pp. 1–3.

Health Care Financing Administration. *Profile of Medicare, 1988.* Washington, D. C.: Health Care Financing Administration, 1998.

Heiss, F.; McFadden, D.; and J. Winter. Who Failed to Enroll in Medicare Part D, and Why? Early Results. *Health Affairs Web Exclusive*, 344–354, 2006.

Himmelfarb, R. *Catastrophic Politics: The Rise and Fall of the Medicare Catastrophic Coverage Act of 1998.* University Park, Pa: Pennsylvania State University Press, 1995.

Historical Background and Development of Social Security, http://www.ssa.gov/history/briefhistory3.html, 2009.

Holahan, John and Alshadye Yemane. Enrollment is Driving Medicaid Costs—But Two Targets Can Yield Savings. *Health Affairs* 28(5): 1453–1465, 2009.

Hsiao, W. C.; Yntema, D. B.; Braun, P.; and E. Becker. Resource Based Relative Values: An Overview. *Journal of the American Medical Association* 260: 2347–2353, 1988.

Hsiao, William C. Objective Research and Physician Payment: A Response from Harvard. *Health Affairs* 8(4): 72–75, 1989.

Hyman, David A. *Medicare Meets Miphistopheles.* Washington, D.C.: Cato Institute, 2006.

Jaffe. S. *Competitive Bidding in Medicare Advantage.* Robert Wood Johnson Foundation. 2009. http://www.rwjf.org/healthreform/product.jsp?id=43710.

Kahn, Charles N., III. Payment Reform Alone Will Not Transform Health Care Delivery. *Health Affairs* 28(2): w216–w218, 2009.

Kaiser Family Foundation. *Medicare Advantage, Fact Sheet.* April, 2009. http://www.kff.org/medicare/upload/2052-12.pdf.

Kaiser Family Foundation, Kaiser Commission on Medicaid and the Uninsured. *Health Coverage for Low-income Children.* January 2007. http://www.kff.org/uninsured/upload/2144-05.pdf.

Kemper, Peter and Christopher M. Murtaugh. Lifetime Use of Nursing Home Care. *New England Journal of Medicine.* 324(9): 595–600, 1991.

Koch, Alma, L. Financing Health Services. In Stephen J. Williams and Paul R. Torrens (Eds.). *Introduction to Health Services.* pp. 335–370. New York: John Wiley, 1988.

Kotlikoff, Laurence J. *The Healthcare Fix: Universal Insurance for all Americans.* Cambridge, MA: Massachusetts Institute of Technology Press, 2007.

Kronenfeld, Jennie Jacobs. *Expansion of Publicly Funded Health Insurance in the United States: The Children's Health Insurance Program and Its Implications.* Lanham, MD: Lexington Books, 2006.

Kronenfeld, Jennie Jacobs. *Health Care Policy: Issues and Trends.* Westport, CT: Praeger, 2002.

Kronenfeld, Jennie Jacobs and Michael R. Kronenfeld. *Healthcare Reform in America: A Reference Handbook.* Santa Barbara, CA: ABC-CLIO, 2004.

Landon, B. E.; Zaslavsky, A. M.; Bernard, S. L.; Cioffi, M. J.; and P. D. Cleary. Comparison of performance of traditional Medicare vs. Medicare managed care. *Journal of the American Medical Association* 291(14), 1744–1752, 2004.

Laugesen, Miriam J. Siren Song: Physicians, Congress and Medicare Fees. *Journal of Health Politics, Policy, and Law* 34(2): 157–179, 2009.

Lee, Christopher. Social Security, Medicare Panel Adjusts Forecasts. *Washington Post.* April 24, 2007. http://www.washingtonpost.com/wp-yn/content/article/2007/04/23/AR2007042301963.html.

Letch, Suzanne W. et al., National Health Expenditures, 1991. *Health Care Financing Review.* (Winter, 1–30), 1991.

The Long-term Outlook for Medicare, Medicaid, and Total Health Care Spending. 2008. http://www.cbo.gov/ftpdocs/102xx/doc10297/Chapter2.5.1.shtml.

Marmor, Theodore R. *The Politics of Medicare.* 2nd Ed. New York: Aldine de Gruyter, 2000.

Mayes, Rick and Robert A. Berenson. *Medicare Prospective Payment and the Shaping of U.S. Health Care.* Baltimore, MD: The Johns Hopkins University Press, 2006.

McFadden, Daniel. An Evaluation of Medicare Part D. *Economist's Views.* February 16, 2007. http://www.typepad.com/services/trackback/6a00d83451b33869e200d8351a332c69e2.

McIlrath, Sharon. HCFA Issues Final RBRVS Rules. *American Medical News,* pp. 1, 26, and 47, 1991b.

McIlrath, Sharon. RBRVS Launch Could Be Difficult. *American Medical News,* pp. 1–37, December, 1991a.

Medicare and Long-term Care Factsheet. Georgetown University Long-term Care Financing Project. February, 2007. http://ltc.georgetown.edu/pdfs/medicare0207.pdf.

Miller, R. H. and H. S. Luft. Managed care plan performance since 1980. A literature analysis. *Journal of the American Medical Association* 271(19), 1512–1519, 1994.

Moon, Marilyn. *Medicare Now and In the Future.* Washington, D.C., Urban Institute Press, 1993.

Moran, M. Managed care's unfulfilled promise: Making prevention part of the medical culture requires a change of values. Progress is coming, but slowly. *Amednews.com,* February 1, 1999. http://www.ama-assn.org/amednews/1999/pick_99/feat0201.htm.

Morgan, Paulette C. and Madeline Smith. Medicare + Choice: Private Fee-For-Service Plans. In Colamery, S. N., (Ed.) *Medicare: Current Issues and Background.* New York, Nova Science Publishers, Inc., 2003.

Morgan, Paulette C.; Smith, Madeline; and Hinda Ripps. Chaikind. Medicare + Choice: Plans Leaving the Program. In Colamery, S. N., (Ed.). *Medicare: Current Issues and Background.* New York, Nova Science Publishers, Inc., 2003.

Morone, James A. American Political Culture and the Search for Lessons from Abroad. *Journal of Health Politics, Policy, and Law 15* (Spring), 129–143, 1990.

Oberlander, Jonathan. *The Political Life of Medicare*. Chicago, IL: University of Chicago Press, 2003.

O'Brien, Mary Jo; Archdeacon, Meghan; Barrett, Midge; Crow, Sarah; Janicki, Sarah Rousseau, David; and Claudia Williams. *State Experience with Access Issues under Children's Health Insurance Expansions*. New York: Commonwealth Fund, Publication No. 384, 2000.

O'Sullivan, Jennifer; Merck, Carolyn; Smith, Madeline; Tilson, Sibyl; and Heidi G. Yacker. Medicare Reimbursement Policies in *Medicare: Current Issues and Background*. Edited by S. N. Colamery. New York: Nova Science Publishers, 2003

Reinhardt, Uwe E. Does the Aging of the Population Really Drive the Demand for Health Care? *Health Affairs* 22, no. 6: 27–39, 2003.

Rice, Thomas. An Economic Assessment of Health Care Coverage for the Elderly. *Milbank Quarterly* 65(4): 288–520, 1987.

Rice, Thomas and Nelda McCall. The Extent of Ownership and the Characteristics of Medicare Supplemental Policies. *Inquiry* 22 (Summer): 188–200, 1985.

Rodwin, Victor. Physician Payment Reform: Lessons from Abroad. *Health Affairs* 8(4): 76–83, 1989.

Rosenbaum, Sara; Johnson, Kay; Sonosky, Colleen; Markus, Anne; and Chris DeGraw. The Children's Hour: The State Children's Health Insurance Program. *Health Affairs* 17: 75–89, 1998.

Rother, John A. Consumer Perspective on Physician Payment Reform. *Health Affairs* 28(2): w235–w237, 2009.

Rovner, J. Democratic Leaders Slow Pace of Medicare Bill. *Congressional Quarterly Weekly Report* 45(27): 1427–1428.

Schneeweiss, Sebastian; Patrick, Amanda R.; Pedan, Alex; Varasteh, Laleh; Levin, Raisa; Liu, Nan; and William H. Shrank. The Effect of Medicare Part D Coverage on Drug Use and Cost Sharing among Seniors without Prior Drug Benefits. *Health Affairs* 28 (2): w305–w316, 2009. (Published online February, 2009; 10.1377/hlthaff.28.2.w305.)

Schneider, E. C.; Cleary, P. D.; Zaslavsky, A. M.; and A. M. Epstein. Racial Disparity in Influenza Vaccination: Does Managed Care Narrow the Gap between African Americans and Whites? *Journal of the American Medical Association* 286(12): 1455–1460, 2001.

Selden, Thomas M.; Banthin, Jessica S.; and Joel W. Cohen. Medicaid's Problem Children: Eligible but not Enrolled. *Health Affairs* 17: 192–200, 1998.

Shaviro, Daniel. *Who Should Pay for Medicare?* Chicago: University of Chicago Press, 2004.

Stevens, Rosemary. *In Sickness and in Wealth: American Hospitals in the Twentieth Century*. New York: Basic Books, 1989.

U.S. Census Bureau, Population Division, "Projections of the Total Population by Five-Year Age Groups and Sex with Special Age Categories: Middle Series, 1999–2100." Washington: U.S. Census Bureau, January 2000.

Ware, J. E. Jr.; Bayliss, M. S.; Rogers, W. H.; Kosinski, M.; and A. R. Tarlov. Differences in 4-year health outcomes for elderly and poor, chronically ill patients treated in HMO and fee-for-service systems. Results from the Medical Outcomes Study. *Journal of the American Medical Association* 276(13), 1039–1047, 1996.

Weinick, R. M.; Weighers, M. E.; and J. W. Cohen. Children's Health Insurance, Access to Care and Health Status: New Findings. *Health Affairs* 17: 127–136, 1998.

West, Howard. Five Years of Medicare: A Statistical Review. *Social Security Bulletin* 34:17–27, December, 1971.

Wilson, James. *Political Organizations*. New York: Basic Books, 1973.

Wong, H. and F. Hellinger. Conducting Research on the Medicare Market: The Need for Better Data and Methods. *Health Services Research* 36 (1 Part 2), 291–308, 2001.

Xu, K. Tom. Financial Disparities in Prescription Drug Use between Elderly and Nonelderly Americans. *Health Affairs* 22(5): 210–221, 2003.

Zhang, Yuting; Donohue, Julie Marie; Newhouse, Joseph P.; and Judith R. Lave. The Effects of the Coverage Gap on Drug Spending: A Closer Look at Medicare Part D., *Health Affairs* 28(2): w317–w325, 2009. (Published online February 3, 2009;10.1377/hlthaff.28.2.w317.)

INDEX

ABOUT THE AUTHOR

Jennie Jacobs Kronenfeld, PhD, is a professor in the sociology program in the School of Social and Family Dynamics (SSFD) at Arizona State University, Tempe, AZ. Dr. Kronenfeld conducts research in medical sociology, especially in health policy, health across the life course, health behavior, and health-care utilization. She coauthored ABC-CLIO's *Healthcare Reform in America: A Reference Handbook* and authored *Expansion of Publicly Funded Health Insurance in the United States: The Children's Health Insurance Program and Its Implications*. She is the editor of the Emerald Press Research Annual Series "Research in the Sociology of Health Care" and is a past chair of the medical sociology section of the American Sociological Association, and a fellow of the American Academy of Health Behavior.